Living with HHT

A Johns Hopkins Press Health Book

Living with HHT

Understanding and Managing Your Hereditary Hemorrhagic Telangiectasia

Sara Palmer, PhD

Sara Palmer

Johns Hopkins University Press / Baltimore

Note to the Reader: This book is not meant to substitute for medical care, and treatment should not be based solely on its contents. Instead, treatment must be developed in a dialogue between the individual and his or her physician. Our book has been written to help with that dialogue.

Drug dosage: The author and publisher have made reasonable efforts to determine that the selection of drugs discussed in this text conform to the practices of the general medical community. The medications described do not necessarily have specific approval by the US Food and Drug Administration for use in the diseases for which they are recommended. In view of ongoing research, changes in governmental regulation, and the constant flow of information relating to drug therapy and drug reactions, the reader is urged to check the package insert of each drug for any change in indications and dosage and for warnings and precautions. This is particularly important when the recommended agent is a new and/or infrequently used drug.

Johns Hopkins University Press
2715 North Charles Street
Baltimore, Maryland 21218-4363
www.press.jhu.edu

Library of Congress Cataloging-in-Publication Data

Names: Palmer, Sara, author.
Title: Living with HHT : understanding and managing your hereditary
    hemorrhagic telangiectasia / Sara Palmer, Ph.D. .—(A Johns Hopkins Press health book)
Other titles: Living with hereditary hemorrhagic telangiectasia
Description: Baltimore : Johns Hopkins University Press, 2017. | Includes
    bibliographical references and index.
Identifiers: LCCN 2017009942 | ISBN 9781421423906 (pbk. : alk. paper) |
    ISBN 1421423901 (pbk. : alk. paper) | ISBN 9781421423913 (electronic) |
    ISBN142142391X (electronic)
Subjects: LCSH: Hemorrhagic diseases—Genetic aspects—Popular works. |
    Hemorrhagic diseases—Genetic aspects—Treatment.
Classification: LCC RC633 .P35 2017 | DDC 616.1/57042—dc23
    LC record available at https://lccn.loc.gov/2017009942

A catalog record for this book is available from the British Library.

Special discounts are available for bulk purchases of this book. For more information, please contact Special Sales at 410-516-6936 or specialsales@press.jhu.edu.

Johns Hopkins University Press uses environmentally friendly book materials, including recycled text paper that is composed of at least 30 percent post-consumer waste, whenever possible.

To Lev and Suzanne

Contents

Acknowledgments

Many people assisted me in bringing this book to light. Thanks are due first and foremost to Marianne Clancy, executive director of Cure HHT, and Jackie Wehmueller, my editor at Johns Hopkins University Press. They believed in my vision for this book and had confidence in my ability to write it. Their cooperation, enthusiasm, and input on the project from start to finish made the book possible. I am grateful to Marianne for her years of dedicated service to the HHT community, to Jackie for her insightful editing and advice, and to both for their friendship and support.

Lauren Linhard, a communications associate at Cure HHT, was indispensable in connecting me with the HHT community, recruiting interviewees, and collecting consent forms. She cheerfully responded to dozens of e-mails and phone calls. Thank you, Lauren.

Many thanks go to the HHT experts and health care providers whose wisdom improved this book. Dr. Daniel Picus, of Washington University School of Medicine, and Dr. Karel terBrugge, of the University of Toronto, read and commented on the material pertaining to arteriovenous malformations (AVMs) in the lungs and brain and provided essential input on medical and technical details. Dr. terBrugge also contributed the brain images. Ofri Leitner, MS, LCGC, an independent genetics consultant, reviewed the material on the genetics of HHT and provided valuable insights and information. Marianne Clancy's input was important to improving the chapter on research in HHT. Drs. Sally Mitchell and Bernard Cohen, of Johns Hopkins University School of Medicine, contributed the images of lung AVMs and the photographs of skin and mouth telangiectasias. My questions were answered by many HHT physicians, including Drs. Andrew J. White, Raj S. Kasthuri, James Gossage, Mark Chestnut, and Marie Faughnan.

I am deeply grateful to the people who shared their experiences with HHT, including its effects on their health, their emotions, and their family life. Their personal stories give life to the book, demonstrating both the challenges faced by people with HHT and the personal strengths that enable them to cope and to thrive.

Writing can be a lonely business, and I am thankful for the many friends who got me away from my desk for lunches and walks, listened patiently to my endless progress reports, understood my obsession with HHT, and consistently cheered me on.

Last but not least, I am grateful for my wonderful husband, children, and grandchildren. They bring joy to my life every day and fill me with hope for the future.

Living with HHT

Introduction

What in the World Is HHT?

A Brief History of Hereditary Hemorrhagic Telangiectasia

What in the world is HHT? That's the question asked by many newly diagnosed patients, by their families, and, unfortunately, by many primary care physicians who have never heard of this uncommon but not so rare disorder. When I was diagnosed with HHT—tentatively by my local gastroenterologist and definitively after a visit to the Yale HHT Center of Excellence—my highly capable internist was a bit embarrassed that he'd missed the diagnosis. But in all fairness to him, he had had just one lecture in medical school that even *mentioned* HHT, and then only in passing. Even if he'd recognized my frequent nosebleeds as a sign of HHT, he probably wouldn't have realized that nosebleeds were just the tip of the iceberg and that further tests were needed to learn how HHT was affecting my body and increasing my chance of having a stroke or other serious problems.

How HHT Got Its Name

Nosebleeds are the most common and visible symptom of HHT and were the first characteristic of the disease to be identified. Nosebleeds are caused by *telangiectasias* (small tangles of blood vessels in which normal capillaries are absent), which are prone to bleeding (*hemorrhage*). In 1896 the French doctor Henri Jules Louis Marie Rendu recognized telangiectasias and nosebleeds as symptoms of a *hereditary* condition that was different from hemophilia (in hemophilia, bleeding is severe because the blood does not clot properly; in HHT, bleeding results from abnormalities in blood vessels, but the blood clots properly).

Over the next 10 years, reports of the disease by Dr. William Osler in America and Dr. Frederick Parkes Weber in Germany led to the name

Osler-Weber-Rendu Syndrome. Many doctors still recognize the disease by this name, found in old genetics textbooks and medical reports. But *hereditary hemorrhagic telangiectasia*, a term first coined in 1909 by Dr. Frederic Hanes, is the currently accepted medical diagnostic term. The abbreviation HHT is commonly used by both patients and doctors, for obvious reasons.

H=Hereditary (genetic; inherited)

H=Hemorrhagic (causes bleeding)

T=Telangiectasia (abnormal blood vessel)

What's So Bad about HHT?

Since the nineteenth century, many hidden symptoms of HHT have come to light. HHT is not just about nosebleeds. We now know that HHT can cause blood vessel abnormalities not only in the nose but on the skin or in the gastrointestinal tract (GI tract or gut), the lungs, the brain, the liver, or, rarely, the spine. The abnormal blood vessels involve a direct connection between an artery and a vein, where normal capillaries are absent. In the nose, mouth, gut, and skin these malformations are called *telangiectasias*; in the internal organs, they are called *arteriovenous malformations* (AVMs). A variety of medical complications can result from these abnormal vessels, especially if they go unrecognized or untreated. Some of the most serious complications include stroke, brain abscess (infection), heart failure, severe anemia, and death.

Here's the Good News

Along with a better understanding of the dangers and complications of HHT, there has been great progress in the ability to diagnose HHT, prevent complications, and treat many symptoms. One of the major treatment advances in HHT came in the 1970s, when Dr. Robert I. White Jr., an interventional radiologist working at Johns Hopkins Hospital, was studying techniques to stop bleeding in blood vessels damaged by trauma and other causes. One technique Dr. White and others were using involved inserting a detachable balloon into large arteries and veins to stop them from bleeding. As fate would have it, an HHT patient with multiple AVMs in his lungs came to Hopkins, where he was cared for by Dr. Peter Terry, a pulmonologist who has since served on the HHT Foundation's Global Research and Medical Advisory Board. Drs. White and Terry discussed this patient and offered an alternative to surgical removal of a part of the lung, which was the usual treatment at that time: they could use their detachable-balloon technique to block the artery supplying the blood flow to the AVMs. The balloons were placed through a catheter inserted into the patient's thigh and threaded through the blood vessels to the lungs; the whole procedure was guided by x-ray. The procedure was successful, and during the next few years more patients with lung AVMs were treated with the same technique, known as *embolization*.

It turns out that around the same time, similar procedures, using steel coils instead of balloons to plug the arteries, were being done in East Germany and elsewhere in the United States. Since then, a variety of materials have been developed to better close the vessels, the technique has been refined, and the procedure is being used around the world for treating lung AVMs and sometimes brain AVMs as well.

Since that time, much has been learned about the various medical complications of HHT. There is now a *genetic test* for HHT, making diagnosis much easier and more accurate, and there are effective medical imaging techniques to determine whether a person has AVMs in their lungs or brain. Preventive measures have been identified to help people with HHT avoid serious health issues, and there are a wide variety of treatments available for many of the symptoms of HHT. Research continues to expand our understanding of the genetics of HHT, why HHT causes different symptoms in different people, and what triggers the development of abnormal blood vessels. This research helps doctors figure out how to treat HHT more effectively with medications and procedures.

Who Has HHT?

HHT has been identified in every racial and ethnic group. About 1 in 5,000 people has HHT, approximately 1.4 million people worldwide. About 95 percent of people with HHT have nosebleeds, but because other blood vessel abnormalities in HHT are often hidden, causing no symptoms until a sudden stroke or other serious complication occurs, *most people who have HHT do not know they have it*. As you will read in this book, many serious complications are completely preventable, and others are quite manageable, if you know you have HHT and you learn what to do about it. This book is intended to teach you everything you need to know so that you can get the best care possible for yourself and your family members with HHT.

The Wind beneath Our Wings: The HHT Foundation International

You may be wondering how all these advances in HHT came about. After all, it's an uncommon disease, and most people—including most doctors—have never heard of it. The answer is simply this: the HHT Foundation International (now called Cure HHT), a nonprofit organization dedicated to supporting and educating people with HHT, teaching doctors about HHT, raising awareness, funding research, and promoting excellence in treatment.

The idea of starting a Foundation for HHT followed Dr. White's early treatment successes with lung AVMs caused by HHT. He imagined a foundation that would help doctors learn more about HHT and help patients find the best treatment. In 1990, he met with another physician, an interested patient, an attorney, and a representative of the National Organization for Rare Diseases to discuss the formation of an HHT foundation. And the following year, fifteen patients and their families met in New Haven, Connecticut (Dr. White was then working at Yale University), for the first organizational meeting of the foundation. The first patient meeting was held in Columbus, Ohio, in 1992, and in 2001 the foundation's board of directors hired an executive director, Marianne Clancy. Marianne still holds this position today, and she remains a passionate and energetic advocate for people with HHT.

After years of nosebleeds, nasal surgery, and watching my 5-year-old recover from a brain hemorrhage, I still didn't know what I had. I happened to look up "nosebleeds" on the Internet one day, and was directed to the HHT Foundation website. All was now clear! I took the information from the website to my GP, who referred me to a specialty center where my diagnosis was confirmed. My children and I have been treated for lung AVMs and I am taking medicine for my nosebleeds, which have become less severe.   —*Toby**

From the beginning, the HHT Foundation has offered practical information and emotional support for patients and families with HHT. Trish Linke, one of the foundation's original board members, started the first HHT newsletter, *Direct Connection*. Trish, who passed away in 2015, answered calls and provided empathy, information, guidance, and referrals. As technology evolved, Trish designed and moderated the HHT Message Forum; later she answered questions and commented on posts on the Cure HHT Facebook page. Other staff members have taken over these roles, and Cure HHT continues to be a source of information and support for people with HHT. Along with saving lives by connecting patients with doctors who can help them, Cure HHT is an emotional lifeline for countless patients. No one is turned away, and all e-mails and phone calls are answered by human beings.

Initially running on a shoestring budget with very few staff, the foundation raised funds for HHT research, educated patients and doctors around the world, and launched a program of certification for HHT Centers of Excellence, where patients could be treated by doctors who had experience in HHT. The first center was at Yale University, and as of this writing there are twenty-five centers in North America and twenty-two in other locations around the world.

Grass-roots fundraising allowed the HHT Foundation to award research grants that jump-started and sustained quality research on HHT during the many years before scientists were able to obtain federal funding for this uncommon disease. In 2015 the foundation funded six research projects with a total of $230,000, the largest amount in its history. This included special research grants to support innovative projects by young scientists; two scientists who received these small grants from the foundation have since been awarded million-dollar grants from the National Institutes of Health (NIH)

* To protect their privacy, the people whose stories appear in this book are identified by pseudonyms. Some stories are composites of several people's experiences or are fictionalized examples of experiences common to many people with HHT.

to continue their promising work on the genetics of HHT. The foundation has also been instrumental in developing the HHT Outcomes Registry, which will allow scientists to conduct clinical research studies and develop new therapies for HHT.

Cure HHT organizes regional and national education conferences for patients and families at which doctors, researchers, and other health professionals share the latest treatment options, bring patients up to date on research studies, and present information on insurance coverage for HHT, psychological aspects of HHT, and other relevant topics. The foundation also holds scientific conferences every other year. At these conferences, professionals present their latest research results and treatment innovations, exchange ideas, and forge collaborations.

The HHT Foundation/Cure HHT is the one resource that patients and families can count on for up-to-the-minute information on HHT and emotional support in dealing with a new diagnosis or a medical complication. That's why I call it "the wind beneath our wings." I turned to the HHT Foundation when I was first struggling to understand the meaning of my diagnosis, and it pointed me to the HHT Center of Excellence at Yale University. The rest, as they say, is history.

My HHT Story

Among my earliest memories is staying over at my grandparents' apartment at age 3. As I bent over to reach for a toy, blood suddenly spilled from my nose. My Nana didn't know this, but I had nosebleeds several times a week at home. Only her reaction made this one memorable for me—she screamed and then ran for cold towels and tissues. When the nosebleed continued, she was ready to call an ambulance until I said matter-of-factly, "Don't worry Nana, this happens all the time." The nosebleed stopped within about five minutes, and we moved on to my bedtime story.

My spontaneous nosebleeds continued throughout my childhood. Nosebleeds in my sleep left my pillowcase stained most mornings, and minor bumps on the nose could set off severe bleeding. When my nose bled at school, teachers told me to lie down or hang my head over the sink, but this only made it worse. Through trial and error, I learned to stop the bleeding myself by applying pressure to my nose.

My parents were worried, but my pediatrician said that nosebleeds in kids were common and I would "outgrow them." In my teens, my nosebleeds decreased, only to start again in my twenties; during my first pregnancy they worsened dramatically. When my first son was born, I took maternity leave but remained unusually exhausted. I returned to work part time, pushing through my fatigue. Two years later, my second son was born. Although I seemed healthy, my fatigue worsened, until staying alert through dinner-time became a real struggle. Soon I was dragging myself through the day, practically numb with fatigue. Yet I never suspected a serious medical condition—I thought all working moms felt this way.

The cause of my fatigue was discovered accidentally when routine blood tests for a minor medical problem unrelated to HHT showed me to be severely anemic. With iron supplements my energy increased, but when I stopped taking iron, I became anemic and exhausted again. After several years, I found a doctor who was determined to get to the root of the problem. He suspected that gastrointestinal (GI) bleeding was causing my anemia and quickly sent me to a specialist. Fortunately, the GI specialist had recently read an article about HHT and remembered that nosebleeds were a common symptom, along with red spots on the skin and mouth. He took my history, examined my lips and tongue, and announced, "I know what you have!" He gave me the article about HHT and suggested I contact the HHT Foundation. Meanwhile, he did a colonoscopy, which showed no bleeding in my gut. He concluded that my nosebleeds alone were the cause of my anemia. I went back on iron supplements and have been taking them ever since.

I must admit that like most people with HHT, I went through a period of denial, putting off my call to the HHT Foundation. I felt so much better once I was taking the iron consistently, and I had no other symptoms. So how bad could it be? But after learning about the serious complications of HHT, I got scared. My younger son was having frequent nosebleeds, and I realized that if I had HHT, he probably did too.

The HHT Foundation referred me to Dr. Robert White at Yale University, where my younger son and I were screened for lung and brain AVMs. Fortunately, neither of us had brain AVMs, but I had one lung AVM, which Dr. White treated with embolization. My older son was also screened but did not have HHT. My mother, symptom free at the time, was screened, and sure enough, she had tiny lung AVMs, confirming her HHT diagnosis.

Several years later, I had the newly available genetic test for HHT, which made it possible for my brother (and later my grandchildren) to be screened with a blood test. Since my brother did not have the gene for HHT, there was no need for additional screenings, and we could stop worrying about him and his children. My mother developed severe GI bleeding from HHT in her seventies, requiring numerous blood transfusions before her death at age 80. My son, now a father of two, has stayed well despite frequent nosebleeds. I've had two additional procedures for lung AVMs, performed at Johns Hopkins Hospital's HHT Center of Excellence. My anemia is stable, and my energy is much improved.

Why I Wrote This Book

I consider myself extremely fortunate to have been diagnosed and treated before experiencing devastating consequences of HHT. But I know that my luck was just that—if I hadn't been referred to a doctor who just happened to have read one article about HHT, I might have had a stroke or brain abscess before my diagnosis. We have a long way to go before most doctors recognize HHT and everyone with HHT is properly diagnosed and receives the proper treatment and preventive measures. Education is crucial to helping both doctors and patients identify HHT and know what to do about it. And that's why I decided to write this book.

In addition to having HHT, I am a rehabilitation psychologist, so I've spent my career helping people who have physical disabilities and chronic illnesses to cope better and live more satisfying lives. Over the last 15 years, I've devoted more of my time to writing. In addition to book chapters and articles for professionals, I've coauthored three books for patients and families about how to live a full life while dealing with various disabilities, including spinal cord injury and stroke. My last book focused on how parents can raise resilient children when one of their children has a physical disability.

As I became more involved in volunteering with the HHT Foundation, I realized that I could apply my professional experience to helping people cope with the emotional and social aspects of HHT. So I began presenting talks and workshops about this at regional and then national HHT family conferences. I created a webinar on the topic and wrote several fact sheets for adults and children on how to live better with HHT (available on the Cure HHT website). Writing a book about HHT seemed like the natural next step—one that would bring together my experience as a psychologist, a writer, a volunteer, and a person with HHT.

How This Book Can Help You and Your Family

While Cure HHT offers a wealth of information and educational opportunities, it may take some poking around to find everything you need. If you're just getting started on your HHT search, you might feel a bit overwhelmed, and you might not understand all the medical information. This book brings together all the basic information you need to understand how HHT can affect your body, what to do about various symptoms, where to get treatment, and how to keep your family healthy. It explains complicated medical information in language that a person with no medical training can comprehend, and it contains a glossary of medical terms to help you understand journal articles or what your doctor has told you about your condition.

In addition, this book deals with HHT's emotional and social effects, such as stress, depression, and grief, and the impact of health problems on work life and family relationships. You can use the information in this book to recognize symptoms of HHT in yourself or a family member; educate your family, friends, or primary care doctor; find a specialized HHT treatment center in your area; learn about treatment options for your particular symptoms of HHT; discover how to screen your children and other family members; find out what you can do to prevent catastrophic health complications; learn to manage stress and relationship problems related to HHT; improve your parenting for children with HHT; learn how to participate in research studies; and access resources for support, patient advocacy, and education in your area.

What's in This Book

While it's most helpful to read the chapters in order, you might want to zero in on a particular chapter that's most relevant to where you are in your HHT journey.

The book is divided into three parts. Part I, "The Many Faces of HHT," comprises three chapters that deal with how HHT is diagnosed, the variety of medical symptoms and complications HHT may cause, how these are treated, and what you can do to prevent some of HHT's most serious complications.

In chapter 1, "Diagnosis: Connecting the Dots," you will learn about the various symptoms of HHT and the medical criteria for making the diagnosis; why it's difficult to make the diagnosis; how a good family medical history can help with the diagnosis; how to confirm the diagnosis with genetic testing and/or clinical screening tests; and where to find doctors with expertise in HHT diagnosis and treatment.

Chapter 2, "The Trouble with Telangiectasias: Nosebleeds, Red Spots, and Bleeding in the Gut," looks at the consequences of telangiectasias, the blood vessel abnormalities in HHT that cause nosebleeds, red spots on the skin and in the mouth (which sometimes bleed), and bleeding in the gastrointestinal tract (gut). Nosebleeds and their management, including prevention, treatment, and coping with emotional stress and social disruptions, are discussed in detail. Telangiectasias on the skin and in the mouth, which are important in diagnosing HHT, are described and illustrated. In addition, the chapter deals with treatments for telangiectasias in the gut and complications of bleeding (from the nose or gut), including iron deficiency and anemia, and how these can be managed to improve health and quality of life.

Chapter 3, "Hidden Dangers: All about AVMs," looks at potential complications of AVMs in the lungs, brain, liver, and spine. It discusses screening, treatment, and preventive measures for AVMs in the lungs and brain, including how recommendations differ for adults and for children. The rare but potentially serious consequences of liver AVMs, treatments for these complications, and the potential of some tests and procedures to make liver AVMs worse are discussed. Finally, the chapter explores less common syndromes in HHT, such as spinal AVMs, pulmonary hypertension, and juvenile polyposis.

Part II, "Living Well with HHT," focuses on how to manage symptoms of HHT to reduce their impact on daily activities, work, emotions, and family relationships and how to promote a better life for people with HHT through advocacy.

In chapter 4, "Taking Care of Yourself: HHT and Your Emotional Health," you will find tips for managing physical limitations and disabilities caused by complications of HHT, including how to plan for your long-term care and options for disability benefits. You will learn about emotional coping strategies to deal with grief, depression, and anxiety and about when to seek professional help for mental health issues.

Chapter 5, "Taking Care of Your Family: Relating to Parents and Siblings and Raising the Next Generation with HHT," addresses the challenges of telling your family about HHT; dating and talking to your partner about HHT; reproductive options and becoming a parent with HHT; teaching your children about HHT; and being a caregiver for your family member who has HHT.

In chapter 6, "Beyond the Family: Conquering Obstacles with Advocacy," the potential benefits of becoming involved in HHT advocacy are discussed, and suggestions are given for advocating in the areas of insurance coverage and medical care, legislative action, awareness, and fundraising.

Part III, "Into the Future," contains a single chapter. Chapter 7, "Frontiers in HHT Research: Expanding Knowledge and Developing New Treatments," describes progress made in HHT care as a result of past research, including basic science and clinical research. It describes new and ongoing HHT research studies and the development of patient registries and databases and discusses the potential for research and data collection to greatly increase our understanding of how HHT works and ways to treat—and someday cure—it. It describes how people may choose to get involved in research by becoming a subject in a clinical trial or other research study or allowing your medical information to be included in a research data base. The chapter looks at how research is funded and provides suggestions on how you can help support research through fundraising and legislative efforts. It ends with final remarks on the future of HHT.

An HHT glossary includes medical and technical terms used in this book as well as terms you might come across in your readings and discussions about HHT. Finally, a section titled "Resources" lists state, national, and international resources for education, support, treatment, prevention, and research on HHT, as well as mental health resources for coping with chronic illness. Included are articles, books, videos, and webinars on HHT; a listing of HHT Centers of Excellence (by state and country); online support groups for people with HHT; the Cure HHT website, www.curehht.org; genetic counseling resources; and national and mental health / therapist associations.

What's Not in This Book

This book is intended to provide a basic education on HHT—everything you need to know to get on the path toward diagnosis, treatment, and prevention of complications. But this book is a product of its time and cannot possibly include all the treatments or research studies that will no doubt come about after its publication. Because scientific advances and treatment methods for HHT are developing at a rapid pace, you will benefit from checking in frequently with the Cure HHT website, HHT Centers of Excellence, and other reputable sources such as the NIH to stay abreast of the latest research and treatment developments. It is my sincere hope that with this book as your basic reference and with supplemental updates from Cure HHT and your doctors, you and your family will stay as healthy as possible and enjoy a good life with HHT for as long as possible.

Part I

The Many Faces of HHT

Chapter 1

Diagnosis
Connecting the Dots

How Do You Know If You Have HHT?

The sad truth is that most people with HHT don't know they have it. In fact, it's estimated that only about 10–15 percent of people with HHT are diagnosed correctly. Many people with HHT—and some doctors—think it's just a "nosebleed disease." But HHT is much more complicated and potentially serious. Medical experts from around the world have identified the major symptoms and complications of HHT and developed four diagnostic criteria to determine whether a person has HHT. Although most of these symptoms can also occur in people who do not have HHT, the presence of multiple symptoms and/or symptoms in multiple related individuals is unique to HHT.

The Four Diagnostic Criteria for HHT

1. Recurrent and spontaneous nosebleeds, which may be mild to severe
2. Multiple telangiectasias on the skin of the hands, lips, or face or inside the nose or mouth
3. Arteriovenous malformations (AVMs) or telangiectasias in the lungs, brain, liver, intestines, stomach, or spinal cord
4. A family history of a first-degree relative (such as a parent, sibling, or child) who meets these same criteria for definite HHT or has been genetically diagnosed

---

A person must have three of the four criteria listed above for a *definite* diagnosis to be made, while HHT is *possible* in those having at least two. To make the diagnosis, doctors need to look at the patient's symptoms and family history; in addition, screening tests are often required to determine whether there are blood vessel abnormalities in the brain or lungs.

The *visible* symptoms of HHT include nosebleeds and telangiectasias of the skin. Abnormal blood vessels (telangiectasias) in the nose are the cause of nosebleeds, the most common symptom of HHT. Almost all people with HHT have nosebleeds by midlife. Frequent or severe nosebleeds may lead to anemia and the need for blood transfusions. Telangiectasias can also occur on the skin, most commonly on the lips, face, hands, and trunk. These appear as red spots and may be a cosmetic concern. Sometimes these telangiectasias bleed.

Invisible blood vessel abnormalities caused by HHT—telangiectasias inside the gastrointestinal (GI) tract and arteriovenous malformations (AVMs) in various internal organs—can result in serious health problems if undetected or untreated. Telangiectasias can occur in the lining of the GI tract, including the stomach and intestines. Like telangiectasias in the nose, they may cause bleeding that ranges from intermittent and mild to frequent and severe. GI bleeding can lead to anemia and the need for blood transfusions.

An arteriovenous malformation is a larger version of a telangiectasia, an abnormal connection between a vein and an artery. AVMs can occur in the brain, the lungs, the liver, or, rarely, the spine. AVMs in the brain carry the risk of brain hemorrhage (bleeding), which can cause brain damage. Potential complications from AVMs in the lungs include bleeding into the lungs, stroke, and brain abscess. In the liver, AVMs can lead to liver and heart failure, although this is rare. And in the spine, AVMs can cause weakness or paralysis.

Finally, family history is critical to diagnosing HHT. HHT is a genetic (inherited) disorder. If your parent has HHT, you have a 50 percent chance of inheriting the disorder. The diagnosis of HHT can be made by genetic testing, but the genetic test does not determine which symptoms of HHT a person will have.

Why HHT Is Hard to Diagnosis

Most Doctors Are Unfamiliar with HHT

In my lifetime so far, there has only been one great doctor who diagnosed me in my early twenties and actually knew anything about HHT.
                                                              —*Rachel*

Although my father had HHT with nosebleeds and I began experiencing nosebleeds in my late teens, the full extent of my AVM pathology went undiagnosed for years.   —Joe

If HHT experts know so much, why does it take so long to get diagnosed? One reason is that because it's an uncommon disease, doctors who don't specialize in HHT know very little about it. For a doctor to make the diagnosis, he or she must know enough about HHT to even think of it as a possibility, and then he or she must know which questions to ask and which tests to perform to confirm the diagnosis. In short, the doctor must be able to connect the dots between various symptoms or complications in order to see the full picture of HHT.

Marty was a healthy, active young man until one day a sudden, terrible headache sent him to the hospital. He was diagnosed with a brain abscess and had multiple brain surgeries to treat the infection and relieve swelling in his brain. But the *cause* of the abscess was a mystery. A few days later, Marty had a kidney scan for an unrelated symptom. A part of his lung happened to show up on the kidney scan, and something in the image looked abnormal. So his doctor ordered a CT scan of his lungs and found several AVMs. At this point, Marty's weekly bloody noses came into the conversation . . . and they determined he had HHT. The abscess was caused by bacteria entering his bloodstream through a pulmonary AVM.   —Karen, Marty's fiancée

In Marty's case, the "dots" were connected by the accidental finding of lung AVMs. This revealed the source of Marty's brain abscess (bacteria getting through the AVM in his lung and traveling to his brain) and—because most people with lung AVMs have HHT—led his doctor to consider HHT as a possibility. When the doctor learned that Marty had regular nosebleeds, the final dot was connected, clinching the diagnosis.

People with HHT May Not Feel Sick

Another reason that diagnosis is difficult is that many people with HHT do not feel sick and have no reason to seek medical care. Some people have only the invisible manifestations of HHT, and these may not cause trouble for many decades, if ever. They may feel fine, go to work, raise children, and never know that they have a genetic disorder. Other people with HHT have nosebleeds but view them as normal or adapt to anemia or low oxygen levels and never suspect that they are ill.

> I had a chest x-ray as part of preliminary testing for elective bladder surgery. The radiologist noticed right away that there was something wrong with my lungs. I had four large AVMs, and they suspected I had a rare genetic disorder. At the hospital, my blood oxygen level was 86 percent, and I knew this was a bad reading. The doctor explained that my body had adapted to the low oxygen level and it was like living on a really high mountain top. As he took my family history, it became very clear . . . my mother had died from complications of HHT.
> —*Nina*

Sometimes, as in Nina's case, an unrelated medical problem leads accidentally to the discovery of HHT. Nina might never have known about the lung AVMs if she hadn't needed a preoperative chest x-ray. The AVMs led to a suspicion of HHT, but it was the connection between her AVMs and her mother's history of HHT that led the doctor to make the definitive diagnosis.

HHT Looks Different in Different People

> For as long as I can remember, my mother and several aunts, uncles, and cousins had nosebleeds. When I was a baby, my 14-year-old sister died suddenly in my father's arms. Her death was attributed to "walking pneumonia." Five years later, my brother had a "spot on his lung." He went through a several-hour operation to remove a section of lung containing a blood vessel malformation. When I was 12, my mother suffered a stroke and could not speak when I got home from school.
> —*Donna*

Diagnosis is also difficult because HHT's symptoms vary from person to person. Even among blood relatives, as Donna's story shows, individuals can have very different symptoms of HHT. In another family, for example, a mother and one of three children might have occasional nosebleeds but otherwise feel fine. When the mother's sister, who does *not* have nosebleeds, has an unexplained stroke at age 37, at first there might seem to be no reason to think her stroke is connected in any way to nosebleeds in her relatives. These two sisters might have an elderly uncle who suffers from chronic anemia and a young cousin who experiences shortness of breath during exercise. But how would they know that these are symptoms of the same disease? And how would a doctor seeing just one individual's symptoms know? As in the story of the blind men and the elephant, each doctor diagnoses a different disease, because each sees only the symptoms of one person. But if doctors are aware of the symptoms experienced by multiple family members, they may be able to see a pattern of symptoms and make the connections that the family members could not.

> In seventh-grade reading class I look down at my book and out of nowhere blood drips furiously onto the pages and my tan shirt. Just another "family nosebleed" my mom and I frequently have. My grandmother and her father had them too. My mom has taught me to just hold my head back and wait for it to stop. I'm used to it. Fast forward to life with three children. My 1-year-old daughter wakes up with blood smeared all over her face and hands. Most parents would be horrified at the sight of their little girl looking like this, but I just laughed, snapped a picture, and dismissed it as one of those "family nosebleeds." I'd had surgeries on my nose for frequent nosebleeds, and when my family moved to a new state, I had to find a new ENT doctor. This one had actually heard of HHT—he pulled out his medical text and we read about it together in his office. He joked that he knew I'd go home and Google it, which I did, and the pieces all fit together like a puzzle . . . my mom's and grandmother's nosebleeds they'd always shrugged off . . . my great-grandfather's death due to a brain hemorrhage . . . no one had ever connected it as actually meaning something.
>
> —Lorna

Lorna's new doctor was able to make the diagnosis of HHT after learning that there was a history of frequent nosebleeds in her family—in five generations at least. After reading more about HHT, Lorna herself made the final connection: her great-grandfather's brain hemorrhage. This piece of family medical history could have led to an earlier diagnosis of HHT in Lorna's family.

HHT Mimics Other Illnesses

Diagnosis of HHT is also complicated by the fact that symptoms of HHT can be attributed to other disorders, so the person with the symptom is misdiagnosed, an adequate investigation is not done, and related symptoms or family history never come to light.

> When my daughter was 4 months old, she had her first "asthma" episode. I took her to the hospital, where she received a breathing treatment for oxygen levels in the low eighties. The hospital didn't think much of her numbers, saying that since the equipment wasn't made for babies, it wasn't accurate. In the next year and a half she had quite a few more asthma episodes, each time with readings in the low eighties, and every time the hospital blew it off.   —Connie

Children or adults with breathing difficulties like those experienced by Connie's baby may be misdiagnosed with asthma. Once that happens, the doctor may not look for other causes, such as an AVM in the lungs or anemia from loss of blood in the gut. Similarly, doctors are not likely to order brain images for headaches that look like "ordinary migraines," so the real cause—an AVM or abscess in the brain—goes undetected. Sometimes an AVM in the lung or brain is diagnosed and treated, but because these can occur sporadically in people without HHT, a doctor who's unfamiliar with HHT will not investigate to determine whether this could be the cause.

> I had a great doctor with a wonderful ability to fix lung AVMs but without knowledge of the disease—HHT—that often accompanies them.   —Tanya

Denial: "What I Don't Know Can't Hurt Me"

Finally, confirmation of an HHT diagnosis can be delayed, sometimes with tragic results, because of denial. In individuals with suspected or tentatively diagnosed HHT, it's very common for them to put off getting all the screening tests for lung and brain AVMs, thereby leaving themselves at risk, and/or for family members to refuse to get tested or screened for HHT. Some families may tell themselves, "We only have nosebleeds" or "We've had

three generations with lung AVMs, but we never get HHT in the brain"—
until a grandchild in the fourth generation is born with a brain AVM. And
some people believe that if they don't have any symptoms, they aren't at
any risk. But this is *not* the case. HHT is often invisible and potentially life
threatening. While denial is a common psychological coping mechanism
that helps protect against overwhelming anxiety, denial about HHT can be
very dangerous.

Seeing the Big Picture

For both Marty and Lorna, the diagnosis of HHT explained the cause of
previously mysterious medical events in their families. They learned that
undiscovered AVMs could cause big medical problems if not treated.
Marty's grandmother is a case in point. When she was screened for lung
and brain AVMs after Marty's diagnosis, lung scans revealed several
AVMs big enough to require treatment. Marty's mother had died of a
stroke in her fifties; in retrospect, it was likely that this too had been
caused by HHT—another dot that hadn't been connected to anything at
the time.

> After our baby's stroke, my family put our heads together and made
> the connection between our history of nosebleeds, the sudden death
> of my uncle at age 30, and the brain hemorrhage that my cousin had
> treated five years ago. We're so grateful that our little boy survived
> and is now on the path to recovery. Just a few months after his stroke,
> everyone in our family was screened for HHT, and we found out that
> our 6-year-old has it, I have it, and four of our extended family
> members are also affected.   —*Mike*

For many people with HHT, nosebleeds are an "obvious" symptom of
something but are never linked to other symptoms in the same person or
in his family members until a major complication occurs. Fortunately, recent awareness and education efforts, along with the proliferation of HHT
Centers of Excellence, have been gradually changing that state of affairs.
With better care, education, and support, families can pull together after
an HHT diagnosis, get everyone tested, and reduce their risk for medical
complications.

Compiling Your Own Medical History

If you are reading this book, you probably know or suspect that you or a loved one has HHT. There are a couple of things that can help you or your doctor make a diagnosis. First, take an inventory of *your own* symptoms and medical history; second, gather information about *your family's* medical history. This is especially important if you have moved or changed doctors many times, if you and your primary relatives live in different locations and have different doctors, and/or if you have had only one obvious symptom of HHT (usually nosebleeds).

Here is a list of symptoms or complications that you should include in your personal and family medical history. Note whether *you* or any *family members* (parent, sibling, child, grandparent, or parent's siblings) have experienced them:

- Nosebleeds (at any point in life, of any severity)
- Telangiectasias (red spots) on the lips, face, or fingertips or in the nose or mouth
- Stroke (with no known cause)
- Brain abscess
- Hemorrhage (bleeding) in the lungs
- Hemorrhage (bleeding) in the brain
- Unexplained bleeding in the gut
- Anemia and/or iron deficiency (or the common effects of anemia: shortness of breath, fatigue)
- Liver failure
- Heart failure
- Low blood oxygen levels (or the common effects of this: shortness of breath during exercise, fingertips turning blue)
- Need for blood transfusions

You might know that family members have experienced some of these symptoms, but you probably aren't aware of others. It's a good idea to ask your parents and siblings for information about their medical history and about the medical history of other relatives, such as aunts and uncles, and of past generations. The symptoms of HHT vary widely among related individuals. Maybe your mother had no obvious symptoms but *her* mother did (it's possible that your mother inherited HHT and did not have any complications but passed the gene for HHT on to you). Maybe your mother has no symptoms, but her brother had a stroke at an early age or had a bout with nosebleeds that you've never heard about.

Up, Down, and Sideways: Knowing Where to Look for HHT in Your Family

Once you're diagnosed with HHT, it's essential to begin the process of figuring out which of your family members also have HHT. HHT is always inherited directly from a parent (except in very rare cases where a new, spontaneous mutation occurs), and each child of someone with HHT has a 50 percent chance of inheriting HHT. So looking "up" to your parents, "down" to your children, and "sideways" to your siblings (who share the same 50 percent chance of inheriting it from your parent) is the best strategy to begin with. In some cases, you may easily narrow the search when looking "up," for example, if one parent has nosebleeds or some complication that you now know may have been caused by HHT. If so, that parent can be tested first. But sometimes, as in my family, it isn't easy to tell which of your parents you got it from, so that when you first look "up," you will need to delve into your parents' medical histories, searching for clues.

Neither of my parents had nosebleeds, and both were healthy when I was diagnosed with HHT in my thirties. But when I started asking questions, it turned out that my mother had experienced a brief bout of nosebleeds during her early twenties and had even had her nose cauterized while in college. She had had no reason to tell me about this, since it had been a minor problem and the nosebleeds had disappeared completely after a short time. She had never connected them with *my* nosebleeds, which were so much more frequent and chronic. But when her history of nosebleeds came to light as a possible "dot" in our family picture, my mother agreed to be screened at an HHT Center of Excellence. It turned out that she had several small pulmonary AVMs, confirming her diagnosis of HHT.

Looking "down" to your children is easier, especially if they are under 18, since you can decide whether they get tested for HHT. You know your child's health history from day one, so there's no need to interrogate them. *But remember that even if your child has no symptoms of HHT, he or she might still have the disease.* If you have HHT, it's essential that *all* your children be tested. If one or more of your children has nosebleeds and/or skin telangiectasias, it makes sense to start with them, but your children who are symptom free should also be screened.

If your children are adults, you may face some resistance to getting tested or learning about HHT. Many young adults feel invincible and avoid any preventive medical care. It's best to share with them as much information as possible about HHT and its potential complications and to express your concern about their health, without forcing the issue or creating a battle of wills. Initial resistance to being tested for a disease is common, especially when the person shows no obvious symptoms.

In fact, many people diagnosed with HHT are met with stubborn denial when looking "sideways" to discover whether their siblings have symptoms of HHT and to encourage them to get tested. Even in families that have experienced tragic consequences of HHT, adult siblings may resist getting tested, saying, "I can't handle knowing" or "What I don't know can't hurt me." You may be able to gently chip away at this denial by pointing out that *you* have been able to handle the knowledge of having HHT, that knowing will *protect* them against getting hurt, and that getting tested may help them safeguard the health of their children. Presenting information, resources, and support is the way to go. Avoid getting into a fight or contest with your siblings; try to lead by example and keep the lines of communication open. Enlist your siblings' help in gathering medical information about aunts, uncles, and grandparents; they may start to get the point as they see a pattern of symptoms emerge in your shared family history. And last but not least, offer your parents, children, and siblings a sense of *hope* by emphasizing that diagnosis and treatment can *prevent* strokes and other complications and that many good treatments for HHT are available and more are being developed through ongoing research.

Organizing Your Family's Medical Information

Once you've been able to gather information from your family members, how can you keep track of it all? An easy tool to track, save, and print your family medical history is "My Family Health Portrait," provided by the US Department of Health and Human Services. This free form is available online at https://familyhistory.hhs.gov/FHH/html/index.html. The form can be updated, and you can print it out to share with family members and doctors. Booklets that teach you how to gather a good family health or genetic history and how to approach your family members about this topic are provided free by Genes in Life at http://www.genesinlife.org/order-family-member. (Your primary care provider may also be able to provide you with a good medical history form.) These tools include general health information that goes beyond symptoms or consequences of HHT, such as high blood pressure, cholesterol, diabetes, smoking, allergies, and more. This type of information is important to share with your doctor if you require treatment for any of your HHT symptoms, and it can be useful should you develop a medical problem that's *not* related to HHT.

Several online services allow you to keep your family medical history in a secure server that only you can access. But you can also save this information yourself on your own computer and update it whenever there is a new medical event or a new person is born in your family. And if you aren't a "computer person," you can write down your family's health history in a notebook and keep it in your file cabinet.

What to Do Next: Confirm Your Diagnosis

If you've already gathered your family history, noted all your symptoms, and read up about HHT in this book or elsewhere, you and your doctor may be pretty sure that you have HHT. Next, you need to confirm your diagnosis and find out which of your family members have HHT. This can be done through genetic testing and/or clinical screening tests.

Genetic Testing

My mom and sister could have found out years earlier about their AVMs. They had been needlessly walking around for nearly 10 years with these ticking time bombs in their lungs, and I am so grateful that nothing bad happened. We have since had genetic testing done on the whole family. My son was diagnosed with HHT, as was one of my nephews. My recommendation to family members of people with HHT is to definitely get tested whether you have symptoms or not.
                                                              —*Tanya*

Genetic testing is useful because it can eliminate the need for everyone in a family to be clinically screened for HHT. This saves money, time, and worry over multiple generations. To understand the usefulness and limits of genetic testing, it's helpful to know how HHT is inherited.

Every person has two copies of each gene, one inherited from each parent. HHT is caused by a mutation in genes that affect blood vessel development, resulting in the development of telangiectasias and AVMs in place of normal blood vessels. HHT is *autosomal dominant,* which means that if you get *one* defective copy of the gene, you will have HHT even though your other copy of the gene is normal. Since each person with HHT has one good copy of the gene and one defective copy, he or she has a 50 percent chance of passing the disease on to any of their children. Either the child will get one normal copy of the gene from his parent with HHT (and one normal copy from his parent who does not have HHT) and *not inherit* HHT or the child will get one defective copy from his parent with HHT (and one normal copy from his parent who does not have HHT) and *inherit* HHT (fig. 1.1). HHT does not skip a generation; therefore, if you do not inherit HHT, your children will have no chance of getting it. But if one of your parents has HHT, you and your siblings have a 50 percent chance of having HHT; and if you have HHT, any of your children and any of your siblings have a 50 percent chance of having it too. *These are people who need to be tested for HHT.*

So far, five different genes have been identified as capable of causing HHT, and many different mutations on these genes have been discovered. The three genes identified as causing most cases of HHT are the endoglin (or *ENG*), *ACVRL1* (or *ALK1*), and *SMAD4* genes. The *SMAD4* gene mutation is very rare, occurring in about 2–3 percent of people with HHT. This mutation causes not only HHT but also another disease, juvenile polyposis. Two other genes, *GDF2* and *RASA1*, were recently identified as causing HHT in a small percentage of families.

Who Should Get the Genetic Test?

The genetic test is most useful for children, parents, or siblings of a person with definite HHT who do not have obvious symptoms of HHT. Because the genetic test is much easier than clinical screening tests for HHT, family members may be more willing to have the genetic test if it's an option. But that means that someone in the family who has HHT has to go first. Ge-

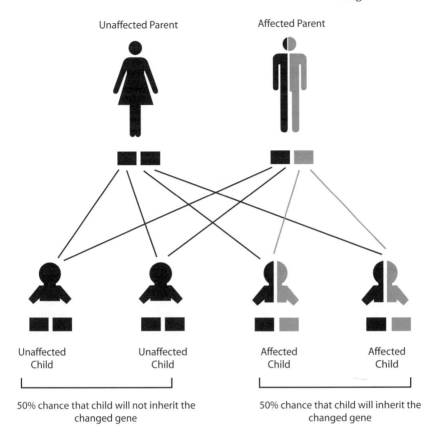

Figure 1.1 Autosomal Dominant Inheritance of HHT

netic testing for a family starts with one person who already has a definite clinical diagnosis of HHT, which makes it possible for that person's relatives—and future generations of their families—to get tested more easily. This phase, called *site-specific testing*, involves a complicated analysis of all three genes known to cause HHT and "reading" the sequences on each gene to discover where it is defective. Many different mutations on these three genes can cause HHT, but once the gene and the particular mutation on that gene are identified, testing of other family members is much easier (and cheaper) because analysis looks only for the mutation that was found in the first person tested.

In about 85 percent of people, genetic testing for HHT can clearly identify a gene mutation and determine whether the person has HHT. If another family member has the same mutation, then he has HHT. If not, he doesn't have it, no further screening is needed, and he cannot pass HHT on to his children or future generations. But in 15 percent of people who have a clinical diagnosis of HHT, genetic testing does not provide a clear answer; no mutation is identified on genetic testing. In those individuals' families, the genetic test is not useful for identifying which family members have inherited HHT, so each person at risk for HHT needs to undergo clinical screening, whether or not he or she has symptoms of HHT. In some people, the genetic testing finds a *variant of uncertain significance*, or *VUS*, which means that there is a change in the gene, but one that is not clearly associated with HHT. Family members of these people must also have clinical screening.

Where to Get Genetic Testing

Genetic testing can be done through a genetics lab that offers the test (see the "Resources" section of this book) or at an HHT Center of Excellence (see below). Your doctor must provide a referral for the testing. If you live far from a genetics lab or hospital that does the testing, you can make arrangements for your local doctor or lab to take your blood sample and send it to the genetics lab by mail. Some labs can do genetic testing with a sample of saliva rather than blood, which makes it easier to test babies and young children.

Clinical Screening for HHT

Clinical screening tests are necessary to discover whether a person has *invisible* symptoms of HHT. These screenings are recommended for people whose diagnosis of HHT is definite based on clinical criteria or genetic testing, as well as for people who have not had genetic testing (or for whom genetic results were inconclusive) but have a possible diagnosis of HHT based on having a child, parent, or sibling with definite HHT. But it's only useful to screen for abnormalities that can be treated to prevent later medical complications. HHT experts agree that *all* people diagnosed with HHT (or at risk for having HHT) should be screened for lung and brain AVMs, because treating these can prevent strokes and brain abscesses. Basic screening tests for lung AVMs are the contrast echocardiogram and computed tomography (CT) scan of the lungs. Basic screening for brain AVMs is done by magnetic resonance imaging (MRI) of the brain. These screening tests, along with treatments for lung and brain AVMs are discussed in detail later in this book.

Where to Get Clinical Screening: HHT Centers of Excellence

The best place to have a thorough evaluation for HHT, including clinical screening, is at an *HHT Center of Excellence (COE)*. An HHT Center of Excellence is a multispecialty medical practice offering comprehensive care to people with HHT. After your evaluation, the center can provide the treatments you and your family need for HHT-related medical problems. The COEs are certified by the HHT Foundation International. They must meet standards of care set by the foundation in consultation with medical experts and advisers. The centers provide clinical experts from a variety of medical specialties who are knowledgeable about HHT. These experts work as a team to take care of the patients seen at the center. A nurse or other patient care coordinator works closely with these physicians to make sure patients get the right screening tests, have appointments with all the doctors they need to see, get proper follow-up care, and are scheduled for treatment procedures when necessary. COE coordinators frequently assist patients with obtaining insurance coverage for their screenings and treatments at the center. The goal of the HHT COE is to provide a "one-stop shopping" experience for people with HHT.

Instead of having to make appointments with an ENT (otolaryngologist), a gastroenterologist, a hematologist, a cardiologist, a pulmonologist, a radiologist, a dermatologist, and possibly other specialists, you can see all of these doctors at an HHT Center of Excellence. There, doctors communicate with one another to develop a coordinated plan for your care. Because of their special expertise in treating HHT patients, they are likely to be up on the latest research studies about HHT and to know which treatments are best for you and when to intervene and when to watch and wait. Most centers have a genetic counselor to help individuals navigate the genetic testing process and discuss options for family planning and prenatal testing.

Your first visit to a COE may take one or two days. When your evaluation is complete, one of the COE doctors will go over your test results, treatment options, and recommendations for follow-up care. You should leave with a much better understanding of how HHT affects you (and/or your family member) and a clear plan for what to do: prevention strategies, further testing, necessary treatments, and recommendations for managing nosebleeds or other symptoms at home.

At the time of this writing, there are 25 HHT Centers of Excellence in North America, as well as many centers in other parts of the world (see the "Resources" section). New centers will be added in the future. An up-to-date list of all HHT centers can be found on the Cure HHT website.

Other Places to Get Treatment

If you live too far from the nearest HHT Center of Excellence and travel is impractical, there may be specialists in your local area to help manage your HHT. While the COEs are the gold standard for HHT treatment, some community physicians are willing to listen to individuals with HHT, communicate with an HHT COE (or with staff of Cure HHT), and educate themselves to apply their specialty skills to the treatment of HHT. In fact, Cure HHT now has a registry of doctors in various specialties and geographic areas who have some familiarity with HHT and are interested in treating patients with HHT.

Once you've been diagnosed and treated, monitoring your health can often be easily handled by your primary care doctor. If a problem is discovered (for example, if you become severely anemic), your doctor can refer you back to an HHT specialist for further study or treatment recommendations. What's essential is that your local doctor is willing to coordinate with HHT specialists so you can get the best care. Providing your doctor with information about your own and your family's HHT symptoms and with educational materials about HHT in general is extremely helpful. Remember to take your medical history printout (or notebook) when you visit any new doctor. It's also helpful to give your doctor basic information about HHT that is written for physicians, such as the fact sheet "HHT Quick Facts for Health Care Professionals," available on the Cure HHT website (see the "Resources" section of this book).

Whenever you visit your local doctor, make sure the HHT Center of Excellence gets a copy of his or her note, and vice versa. The best way to do this is to request a copy of your office visit note and a report of all test results after every appointment, then mail, fax, or e-mail them to your doctor(s) yourself. (Don't depend on the center or your doctor to do the communicating; sometimes things fall through the cracks.) If you have screening tests at your local hospital or radiology center, make sure to request an actual CD of the images and send this to the person at your HHT Center of Excellence who is most expert at interpreting them. If there is any disagreement between your local doctor and your HHT COE doctor about what type of treatment you need (for example, if your MRI shows a brain AVM), you should consider getting another expert opinion; you can do this either by visiting another COE or by mailing your MRI films to another COE and then having a consultation over the phone.

What's Next?

Connecting the dots and discovering that you have HHT can be scary at first. But it can also be a big relief to know that your mysterious symptoms are part of a treatable medical disorder. What's more, you can take an active role in educating your family and protecting your children's health. The knowledge that you have HHT is truly empowering, because now you can do something about it. There's no cure for HHT at this point, and some complications cause unavoidable health problems. Still, once you know you have HHT, most medical complications are either preventable or manageable. The next step is to learn all about the various symptoms and complications of HHT and how to prevent, manage, and treat them so you can stay as healthy as possible.

Chapter 2

The Trouble with Telangiectasias
Nosebleeds, Red Spots, and Bleeding in the Gut

Nosebleeds: HHT's Most Common Symptom

> I have had nosebleeds every day, going back to kindergarten. —*Tom*

> I have had severe nosebleeds since I was 9. I would sometimes faint from nosebleeds lasting more than 20 minutes. —*Joy*

Bleeding from the nose (in medical jargon, *epistaxis*) is by far the most common symptom of HHT. About 95 percent of people with HHT will have some nosebleeds by the time they reach midlife. Although not as potentially dangerous as lung or brain AVMs, nosebleeds frequently disrupt everyday activities and can result in health-threatening or even life-threatening blood loss.

> I had nosebleeds as a child, as did my father and two of my six siblings. At age 12, the bleeding got worse. I had my nose cauterized on countless occasions, without success. At age 19, I had surgery to remove the bleeding areas. Now, at 73 years old, I take medicine for my nosebleeds, which helps the severity but not the frequency.
>
> —*Toby*

In some people, nosebleeds start in adulthood, are occasional or very mild, and may be more of a nuisance than a serious symptom. In others—sometimes even from the same family—nosebleeds may start early in childhood, be more frequent or severe, or result in serious blood loss and *anemia* (low red blood cell count). In many families with HHT, so many relatives experience nosebleeds that the family starts to think of nosebleeds as normal.

Many people without HHT have occasional nosebleeds, especially in childhood, often as the result of dry air, allergies, or minor trauma to the nose. What's different about nosebleeds in HHT is that they are experienced by multiple siblings or across generations, in adults as well as children. If you, your children, and your mother all have nosebleeds, there is good reason to suspect HHT.

Telangiectasias: HHT's Troubling Ts

Telangiectasias are the troublemakers responsible for nosebleeds. A telangiectasia is an abnormal tangle of blood vessels in which the capillaries, the smallest blood vessels, are missing. Normally, the arteries carry blood from the heart to the other organs. The arteries are large near the heart but get smaller and smaller as they branch out, carrying blood to all parts of the body. Eventually these branches form tiny capillaries, where the oxygen is released from the blood so it can fuel the muscles, brain, and all other organs. The blood, now depleted of oxygen, flows from the capillaries into the veins, where it can travel to the heart and lungs to pick up more oxygen. The branching of the vessels allows exchange of oxygen at a lower pressure, so vessels are not stretched or traumatized. But when the capillaries are missing, there is a direct connection between the arteries and veins, resulting in a tangle of bulging vessels (the telangiectasia) whose walls are more likely to break, causing bleeding (fig. 2.1).

Fortunately, telangiectasias in HHT affect only *some* of the vessels in your nose. The size and number of telangiectasias determine how severe your nosebleeds will be. Dry air, trauma, temperature extremes, sneezing, and allergies can increase the tendency to bleed, but telangiectasias can bleed spontaneously and unpredictably. Unfortunately, even if you could say three magic words and get rid of all your telangiectasias right now, some new ones would take their place over time. The cells that make up the *mucous membrane* (the smooth, delicate lining of the nose, mouth, and GI tract) are constantly dying off and being replaced by new cells. With this new tissue come new blood vessels and—you guessed it—new telangiectasias.

NORMAL

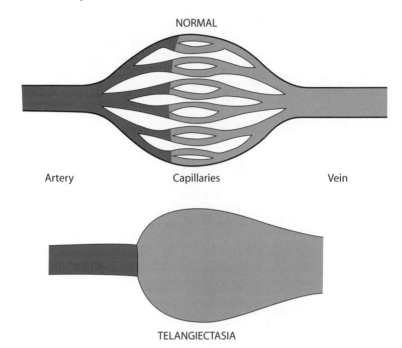

Artery   Capillaries   Vein

TELANGIECTASIA

Figure 2.1 Schematic of a telangiectasia. *Top*, normal capillaries filter the blood and reduce blood pressure in the vessels; *bottom*, abnormal direct connection between an artery and a vein causes shunting of blood to the vein under higher pressure and without filtering. Adapted from Pinar Bayrak-Toydemir, Rong Mao, Susan Lewin, and Jamie McDonald, "Hereditary hemorrhagic telangiectasia: An overview of diagnosis and management in the molecular era for clinicians," *Genetics in Medicine* (2004) 6, 175–191.

Note on Terminology

It's not always clear when to call a vascular malformation in HHT a *telangiectasia* and when to call it an *arteriovenous malformation (AVM)*. Larger abnormalities are usually called AVMs, and smaller ones are called telangiectasias, but these are only relative terms. You may see references to "GI AVMs" in some articles. But more commonly, location in the body, rather than size, determines which term is used. For vascular malformations on the skin and in mucous membranes (nose, mouth, GI tract), the term *telangiectasia* is generally preferred, whereas for malformations in the lungs, brain, and liver the term AVM is preferred. Occasionally, the term *angioectasia* is used for telangiectasias in the gut. The important thing to remember is that *all* these terms refer to the same type of vascular abnormality: a direct connection between an artery and vein in which capillaries are missing. Throughout this book, I use the term *telangiectasia* when talking about these abnormalities in the nose, mouth, or GI tract or on the skin.

Mouth and Skin Telangiectasias

You may recall from chapter 1 that telangiectasias in the mouth and on the skin are another symptom of HHT—and one of the four diagnostic criteria. Telangiectasias in the mouth can appear on the lips, tongue, gums, or soft palate. Some of these are very tiny, flat red dots that are barely noticeable. Some can be larger or raised and appear purplish, like a blood blister.

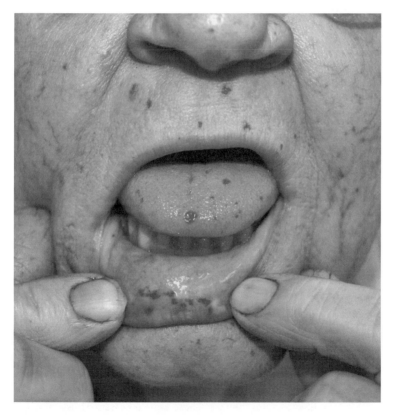

Figure 2.2 Telangiectasias on the lips and tongue. These appear as flat or raised red spots. Photo courtesy of Dr. Bernard Cohen.

These may bleed occasionally, but usually not severely. The number or size of these telangiectasias may increase as a person ages (fig. 2.2).

Telangiectasias on the skin occur mostly on the face and hands (especially on the fingertips) and sometimes on the chest or trunk. These can vary in size from tiny, pinpoint dots to larger, raised areas. They can be round or somewhat spidery. Skin telangiectasias are less prone to bleeding than those in the mouth or nose, but larger telangiectasias on the fingers sometimes bleed, and telangiectasias on the face can be a cosmetic problem (fig. 2.3).

Telangiectasias on the skin or lips can be treated with *laser therapy*, in which a laser light beam heats and destroys the telangiectasias. Laser therapy can also be used on the tongue or palate to treat telangiectasias that cause bleeding. People with HHT tend to get more skin and mouth telangiectasias as they age, but not everyone with HHT will have these characteristic "red spots." One way that telangiectasias differ from the

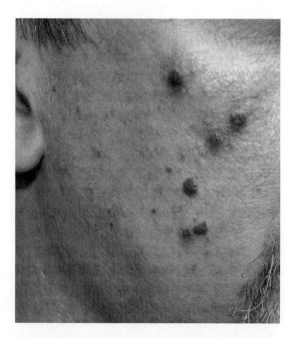

Figure 2.3 Telangiectasias on the face. These appear as flat or raised red spots. Fingertip telangiectasias have a similar appearance. They can vary in size, some are as small as pinpoints. Photo courtesy of Dr. Bernard Cohen.

common, harmless bright red dots that many people get with aging (called *cherry angiomas*) is that if you press on the telangiectasia, it will blanch (turn white), and when you release the pressure, you can see the red color return as the blood flows back into the spot. Many children and adults who do *not* have HHT have some *spider angiomas*, harmless spidery red spots on the skin, or a *few* skin telangiectasias that look just like those in HHT. But the presence of *multiple* telangiectasias on the hands, face, or mouth can be important in diagnosing HHT.

Nosebleed Prevention and Treatment

While telangiectasias on the skin and mouth rarely cause any significant health problems, the same "troublemakers" in the nose are prone to frequent bleeding, which can lead to serious problems related to blood loss. The first line of treatment for these problems (and the best way to avoid the embarrassment and inconvenience of nosebleeds) is to prevent the nose from bleeding in the first place. And many treatments have been developed to prevent or reduce nosebleeds.

Preventing Nosebleeds

The first line of prevention for people with milder nosebleeds is to keep the nose moist. When the lining of the nose is lubricated, the telangiectasias have some protection from dry air or allergens and are less likely to bleed. There are many products for keeping the nose moist, including petroleum jelly, saline sprays or gels, and sesame or other botanical oil preparations. Using a humidifier, especially at night and when air conditioners or heaters are running constantly, will keep the air moist and may reduce nosebleeds.

Beyond moisturizers for the nose, many different substances may have a direct effect on the blood vessels in the nose. *Estrogen cream* applied in the nostrils may make the small blood vessels in the nose stronger and more elastic, but research results have been conflicting regarding its effectiveness. *Tranexamic acid* stabilizes blood clotting and has had good results in several research studies; it is prescribed for some people with moderate to severe nosebleeds. *Bevacizumab* (trade name *Avastin*) inhibits the growth of new blood vessels. Used as a treatment for some types of cancer and, more recently, for bleeding in HHT, it is available as a nasal spray for mild nosebleeds and can also be injected directly into the nasal telangiectasias or given intravenously for moderate to severe nosebleeds. Although more research is needed to prove the effectiveness of Avastin, several smaller studies and reports from clinicians show very good results.

Treating Telangiectasias in the Nose

When the medications named above are not effective or nosebleeds are more severe or prevent a person from participating normally in daily life, there are various procedures aimed at eliminating nasal telangiectasias. One option is *cauterization*, in which the telangiectasias are destroyed with heat. This is usually a short-term solution, because the telangiectasias will grow back over time. Care must be taken to avoid burning healthy tissue or making a hole in the nasal septum (the tissue between the two nostrils), and there is the possibility that repeating the procedure may increase this risk. Chemical cautery (which uses silver nitrate to heat and destroy the telangiectasias) and monopolar electrocautery (a less accurate form of electrocautery) are the procedures most likely to damage the nasal septum and should be avoided. Bipolar electrocautery, in which electricity is passed through the tissue to heat (cauterize) the telangiectasias, uses less heat and carries the least risk of damaging healthy tissues surrounding the telangiectasias.

Another option is *laser therapy*, similar to that used for skin telangiectasias. Laser therapy is relatively safe and can relieve bleeding for 6 to 18 months; some people can have the procedure repeated on a regular basis with success.

Cold ablation (or *coblation*) is a procedure for removing nasal telangiectasias using radiofrequency energy and saline that causes minimal injury to surrounding healthy tissue.

Sclerotherapy is a technique in which an irritating substance is injected into the blood vessels, causing scarring that destroys the telangiectasias. While this has been helpful for some patients, a few have had serious side effects, including a hole in the nasal septum and in one case loss of vision.

In a procedure called *embolization* the flow of blood to telangiectasias in the nose is blocked by inserting tiny particles into the blood vessel through a very small catheter (tube) guided by x-rays. Performed in a hospital under general anesthesia, embolization is rarely recommended except in cases of life-threatening blood loss.

> I faced nosebleeds that were serious enough to send me to the emergency room on more than one occasion. Embolization for my nasal telangiectasias was effective; with good management of my predisposition for nosebleeds, I suffer few and they are mild these days.
>
> —Joe

Septal dermoplasty is a more extreme measure that involves removing the entire nasal mucosa (the layer of tissue lining the nose) and replacing it with a skin graft taken from the patient's leg. Because the mucosa can't regrow once it's removed, this procedure is not reversible. It can be redone, if needed, with additional skin grafting. This procedure is quite effective in preventing nosebleeds, but it requires frequent cleaning and moisturizing of the nose and has unpleasant side effects such as crusting in the nose and an odd smell. It is recommended only for people with *severe* nosebleeds who have not been helped by other treatments.

Another option for people with disabling nosebleeds or life-threatening anemia is *Young's procedure*. This surgical procedure closes the nose completely, so that the person can no longer breathe through the nose. This completely protects the nasal mucosa from irritation due to dry air or particles in the air. Young's procedure dramatically reduces or eliminates nosebleeds and reduces anemia. Side effects include dry mouth (from breathing through the mouth only) and decreased senses of smell and taste. But most people find these side effects preferable to severe, disabling nosebleeds and chronic exhaustion from anemia, and they generally feel better, with improved energy and the ability to reengage in life after the procedure.

> For many years, I needed three or four transfusions a year because of nosebleeds; before my Young's procedure, I needed at least one a month. I had one of the most severe cases of HHT my doctor had ever seen, and the Young's procedure appeared to be the last hope for treating my severe nasal hemorrhaging. After the surgery, the bleeding stopped and I began to regain my strength. I am forever grateful to my doctors.
>
> —Carla

As you can see, there are many treatments to prevent or reduce nose-bleeds. Your HHT doctor can help you decide which treatment is best for you, depending on how severe your nosebleeds are and how they are affecting your health and your daily life. Whether you try some of the over-the-counter moisturizers or oils or another treatment for nosebleeds, it may be helpful to track your progress by calculating your *Epistaxis (Nosebleed) Severity Score (ESS)*; you can do this online at www.curehht.org/living-with -hht/epistaxis-nosebleed-severity-scoring-tool-ess/. After you enter your answers, the score is calculated immediately, and you can print it out for your records and to take to your doctor. Many HHT doctors use this tool to track progress, conduct research, or help make treatment decisions. If you don't have access to a computer, your HHT Center of Excellence can calculate your score.

Epistaxis Severity Score

Please answer the following questions as they pertain to your TYPICAL symptoms WITHIN THE LAST 3 MONTHS for nose bleeding. Please answer all questions.

1. How often do you TYPICALLY have nose bleeding?
   o   Less than once per month
   o   Once per month
   o   Once per week
   o   Several per week
   o   Once per day
   o   Several per day
2. How long does your TYPICAL nose bleeding last?
   o   <1 minute
   o   1–5 minutes
   o   6–15 minutes
   o   16–30 minutes
   o   >30 minutes
3. How would you describe your TYPICAL nose bleeding intensity?
   o   Not typically gushing or pouring
   o   Typically gushing or pouring

4. Have you sought medical attention for your nose bleeding?
   o   No
   o   Yes
5. Are you anemic (low blood counts) currently?
   o   No
   o   Yes
   o   I don't know
6. Have you received a red blood cell transfusion SPECIFICALLY for nose bleeding?
   o   No
   o   Yes

Source: The HHT-ESS was developed by Jeffrey B. Hoag, M.D., M.S. from Drexel University College of Medicine in conjunction with Christian A. Merlo, M.D., M.P.H. and members of the Johns Hopkins University HHT Center of Excellence.

Changes in your ESS score help you see whether your nosebleeds are getting better or worse or staying the same. Depending on your score, you may be a candidate for various treatments or for research studies testing new drugs or procedures.

Managing Your Nosebleeds

> For people with HHT, it is miserable knowing that at the least expected moment—while driving, vacationing, visiting, dancing, eating, relaxing, traveling, or at any time—you can suddenly start bleeding uncontrollably!   —*Rhoda*

How to Stop a Nosebleed

Even if you get your nosebleeds under better control, chances are that you will still have some. So what can you do to manage nosebleeds when they happen? Mild to moderate nosebleeds can usually be managed at home, by yourself or with a little help, as follows:

1. First, sit down and stop whatever you were doing.
2. With a cloth or tissue held against your nose (to catch the drips), put pressure on your nostril(s) for several minutes, leaning your head slightly forward (as if reading a book).

3. *Do not* lean your head back; this will cause the blood to run down your throat, and it will take much longer for the bleeding to stop.

4. It can also be helpful to put an ice cube in your mouth or place an ice pack on your nose.

5. If the bleeding has not stopped after 5 to 10 minutes, continue to apply pressure.

6. *Do not hang your head over the sink and simply let the blood run down the drain.* Although the bleeding will probably stop eventually, this "method" results in more blood loss; you may become dizzy or faint, and it can be frightening to those around you. Applying direct pressure on the nose is likely to be much more effective.

7. Sometimes plugging the nose with a lubricated cotton ball (covered with Vaseline or oil to avoid sticking to the inside of the nose) or a commercial product such as Nasalcease can help stop the bleeding; take care in removing the product so you don't dislodge the clot and start the nose bleeding again.

8. Another method that's helpful for milder nosebleeds is to spray a little oxymetazoline (24-hour decongestant available without prescription) into your nose. Oxymetazoline contains a vasoconstrictor (something that makes the blood vessels contract or shrink) and can help stop bleeding.

For more severe nosebleeds, several types of nasal-packing products are available that you can learn to use at home, including nonstick packing materials, dissolvable packing, and inflatable balloons. Your doctor can help you obtain the right type of packing to use at home. Some types of packing must be done by a doctor in a hospital or clinic.

Make a Plan with Your Doctor

If you've already experienced one or more severe nosebleeds, talk to your doctor about when to treat a nosebleed at home and when to go to an urgent care center or emergency room (ER). If you live near your primary care doctor, you may also have the option of going to his or her office. If you have to go to an ER, remember to tell the doctors you have HHT. Whenever possible, it's best to see a doctor with HHT experience. If your nosebleeds are frequently severe, you should consider one of the treatment options (medication, laser, or surgery) discussed above to help you prevent future emergencies and reduce blood loss.

Plan Ahead

Nosebleeds cause a great deal of stress, largely because they are unpredictable and you never know how long they'll last. While you can't control exactly when your nose will bleed, you can plan ahead so you're prepared to manage a nosebleed when it happens. For example, you can keep tissues in your purses or pockets; identify a friend or family member to call if you need to get help or go to the ER; keep supplies on hand for the home remedies you usually use; and decide in advance where to go for treatment should that be necessary. Some people carry their own customized nosebleed first-aid kit so they can manage nosebleeds whenever and wherever they occur.

Nosebleeds might cause unexpected disruptions in your day, such as being late to work and other appointments. Scheduling time between activities or appointments in case you get a nosebleed can help you stay in control of your schedule and feel less rushed or anxious. Some people may need to limit or change work duties or hours or set aside other activities because of severe nosebleeds and/or the anemia that can result from severe bleeding.

You may notice certain "triggers" for your nosebleeds. Although there is not much research on this, some people report more nosebleeds when they eat particular foods or spices, drink alcoholic beverages, or experience extremes of hot and cold. Avoiding these triggers may be helpful, especially in work or social situations.

Managing the Social Consequences of Nosebleeds

The social consequences of a nosebleed include embarrassment about bleeding on another person or another person's possessions; others' panic or disgust; and the awkwardness of excusing yourself from an important meeting or social event because of a nosebleed. Planning ahead what to say to others about your nosebleeds will help allay their fears. You can say something as simple as, "I have a medical condition that causes nosebleeds, but I'll be OK in a few minutes," or "I'm sorry, but I have a condition that causes unpredictable nosebleeds. I need to excuse myself until it stops." You might want to have a "menu" of requests ready: "I have a medical condition that causes nosebleeds. Can you please call my doctor/call 911/bring me some tissues from the restroom?"

If you bleed on another person, that person might worry about catching HIV or another illness from you. (Some people have wondered whether my nosebleeds were caused by cocaine abuse, which increased their fear that I might have an infectious disease.) If you feel comfortable doing so, you can reassure the person that you don't have HIV or any other blood-borne illness and explain that your nosebleeds are caused by a blood vessel disorder.

I often sniff repeatedly to keep a minor nosebleed from "showing" or to avoid blowing a stuffy nose and causing a bleed. (My ENT's advice was always, "Sniff, don't blow!") People often ask me whether I have a cold. If I feel up to talking about it, I'll tell them about HHT. Otherwise, I just tell them I have allergies so they won't worry about catching anything from me. (While you should never feel obligated to tell strangers details about your medical history, you may find that curiosity about your nosebleeds presents an opportunity for you to educate others about HHT.)

Helping Your Children Manage Their Nosebleeds

> I had nosebleeds since preschool. I always said no to pajama party invitations because I might get a messy nosebleed. Once I said yes to a new girl at school because I really wanted her to like me—but it was a disaster. My nose bled all over the sheets and her mom got hysterical. My dad had to come get me in the middle of the night and I never saw that girl again.
> —*Maria*

Adults who don't know about your child's nosebleeds may become upset about more than the bed linens; they might be afraid of contagious diseases, as discussed above, or they might think they should take your child to the ER. When your child has nosebleeds, it's a good idea to inform the child's friends' parents (and the babysitter, teacher, or any adult who is likely to witness one of the child's nosebleeds) so they won't be frightened. You can give them some basic guidelines so they will know when your child can handle his or her nosebleed and when to call you or get medical help. That said, people tend to be touchy about bloodstains on their things, especially bed linens and clothing. So it's a great help to others if you know how to get rid of the stains. Hydrogen peroxide works on most fabrics without harming them, and many people have it around the house for first aid. Pour a little bit on the stain, let it sit for a few minutes (it will turn white and bubble, which makes it fun for kids to help), and then blot with a clean cloth or cotton pad. If this doesn't completely get the blood out, wash the fabric with soap and *cold* water, rubbing the stain. The quicker you treat the stain, the better, but I've followed this procedure on bloodstains I discovered days after the fact, and it worked fairly well. If your kids with HHT go on a sleepover, send some hydrogen peroxide along in case they bleed on the pillow case. The host parents will be grateful.

Health Problems Resulting from Blood Loss

When treatments for nosebleeds are not effective (or never used), blood loss caused by nosebleeds can lead to serious health problems, including *iron deficiency* (insufficient iron in your body) and *anemia* (insufficient red blood cells in your body). Anemia causes fatigue, shortness of breath, and weakness and may contribute to depression. In severe cases, anemia can lead to heart failure. These symptoms can be disabling, especially if they go untreated. Some people lose so much blood from their noses that they need to have regular blood transfusions.

> I remember seeing my father and grandfather having really bad nosebleeds. Mine didn't get bad until I was in my twenties. When I got my driver's license, I used to take my grandfather "for a fill-up," which is how we referred to his blood transfusions.   *—Arnie*

> On more than one occasion, because of extensive blood loss, my mother's nosebleeds required transfusions.   *—Donna*

Telangiectasias and Blood Loss in the GI Tract

Although less common than telangiectasias in the nose, telangiectasias in the GI tract cause significant bleeding in about 20 percent of people with HHT. (Many others with HHT have GI telangiectasias that do not cause any symptoms or health problems.) This can lead to iron deficiency and eventually to anemia. However, routine screening tests for GI bleeding in people with HHT are *not* recommended. GI telangiectasias don't typically cause significant bleeding until after age 50, and treating asymptomatic telangiectasias in the gut is not advisable because (a) they tend to recur and (b) repeated treatments can cause damage to the wall of the GI tract.

As with nosebleeds, the best defense against blood loss is to reduce or prevent bleeding in the gut with noninvasive medical treatment. Several medicines seem to reduce GI bleeding, but the potential risks and benefits of these drugs have not been proven. Several of the drugs used to treat nosebleeds have also helped some HHT patients with anemia and transfusion dependence because of severe GI bleeding. These include oral estrogen pills, tranexamic acid (Amicar), and bevacizumab (Avastin). However, only a small number of patients have been studied. Larger clinical research studies are needed to show whether Avastin and Amicar are safe and effective for treating GI bleeding.

Thalidomide, a drug involved in blood vessel maturation, was also used in a research study of patients with severe anemia from GI bleeding. While there is evidence that it reduced bleeding, the side effects of the drug, including neuropathy and fatigue, resulted in most subjects' deciding to stop treatment despite the benefits. However, a related drug, pomalidomide, and several other medications are currently being used in research studies to determine their effectiveness in reducing GI bleeding.

In certain circumstances, laser treatment is appropriate and can be effective in reducing GI bleeding. Laser treatment is performed using *endoscopy*, in which a flexible tube with a camera on the end is inserted through the mouth (into the upper GI tract) or the rectum (into the lower GI tract). If telangiectasias are found, they can be destroyed with a laser, just as they are in the nose. Laser treatment for GI bleeding is most effective and least dangerous when there are just a few actively bleeding telangiectasias; eliminating these telangiectasias can reduce the bleeding and improve symptoms of anemia, at least for some period of time. Any laser treatment in the GI tract carries a small risk of perforating the wall of the gut. With repeated or multiple laser treatments, this risk increases substantially, so laser treatment is not recommended when there are many telangiectasias in the gut.

Severe bleeding in HHT, whether from the nose or the GI tract, can be hard to eliminate completely, and even those with less severe bleeding can develop anemia over time. However, the disabling effects of anemia can be reduced with medical management.

Hemoglobin, Iron, and Anemia

Hemoglobin is a protein in red blood cells that carries oxygen through the bloodstream to the tissues. The body uses iron to make this essential protein. But the body cannot make iron, so you have to get it from your food. Normally, the body can store some iron (in the bone marrow, liver, and spleen), but most of the iron is in the hemoglobin, so when you lose blood, you also lose iron. To make up for this *iron deficiency*, the body begins to use its stored iron to make more hemoglobin so that the cells receive enough oxygen. But when the iron stores are used up, the body can't make hemoglobin or replenish the supply of red blood cells, so the tissues can't get enough oxygen. This is called *anemia* or, sometimes, *iron deficiency anemia*, to indicate that loss of iron is the cause. Other medical conditions also cause anemia, but they are beyond the scope of this book.

Symptoms of Iron Deficiency and Anemia

As a boy, I got nosebleeds all the time. When I ran track in high school, I just didn't have as much energy as the other guys on the team. I liked to go hiking in the mountains with my brothers, but I would always poop out way before they were ready to stop.   —*Jamie*

Iron deficiency can cause symptoms before it leads to anemia. In children, iron deficiency can cause difficulties in concentrating, learning, and remembering, as well as difficulty in keeping up with classmates or friends when running or playing sports. In adults, iron deficiency is associated with *restless legs syndrome,* or frequent urges to move the legs or arms because of an uncomfortable feeling.

But most adults (and many children too) develop symptoms only after they have become anemic from lack of iron. These symptoms include fatigue, weakness, headaches, and feeling "winded" or experiencing muscle aches when climbing stairs or performing other strenuous activities. When anemia is severe, fatigue can become disabling, making normal activities like work or household tasks impossible. The exhaustion associated with anemia can contribute to depression or to feeling emotionally "on edge." Severe anemia can cause an *arrhythmia*, a rapid or irregular heartbeat, or *heart failure*, which happens because the heart has to work extra hard to pump more blood to all parts of the body to make up for the lack of oxygen. These heart complications can be fatal if not properly treated.

Diagnosis and Treatment for Iron Deficiency and Anemia

If you have HHT and frequent blood loss from telangiectasias in your nose or GI tract, it's a good idea to get tested for iron deficiency even if you don't have symptoms. If iron deficiency is detected early, you may be able to increase your iron intake and avoid becoming anemic. Of course, if you already have symptoms associated with anemia, it's especially important to get tested. This can be done with routine blood tests, including a complete blood count (CBC), *reticulocyte* (new red blood cell) count, and measures of iron levels in your blood.

There are several common treatments for iron deficiency and iron deficiency anemia. First, there are various ways to replace the iron that is lost from bleeding and replenish the body's stored iron. Iron-rich foods are helpful, but it's difficult to get enough iron from food to replace lost iron stores. Meat, shellfish, and other animal foods contain the form of iron that's easiest for people to absorb; nonmeat sources of iron include soybeans, lentils, and legumes. Most people with iron deficiency related to chronic bleeding need to take *iron supplements*, available over the counter in pill or liquid preparations. Often these supply enough extra iron for the person to recover from anemia. Iron is usually combined with another substance to make it easier to digest and to avoid constipation, a common side effect of iron.

For more severe iron loss, an *iron infusion* may be necessary. This is a liquid preparation of iron that is given intravenously (through a vein), usually at an outpatient medical center. Although there can be some side effects of iron infusion, it is generally safe and painless, except for the slight discomfort of inserting the IV (intravenous) needle. Allergic reactions can be prevented by giving a small test dose before the infusion and pretreating with antihistamine if necessary.

After starting iron supplements, an individual must have repeat blood tests to make sure that his or her iron deficiency or anemia is improving. Depending on one's response to treatment, and whether there is continued regular blood loss, the doctor will advise how much iron is needed and for how long. People with frequent nosebleeds or GI bleeding may need to stay on oral iron supplements for a long time in order to prevent anemia. It is not harmful to take iron supplements for as long as your body continues to need iron.

In the most severe cases of anemia, iron supplements are not sufficient, and a *blood transfusion* may be needed to prevent heart problems and treat symptoms like exhaustion and shortness of breath. People with the most severe GI bleeding are sometimes "transfusion-dependent," requiring a blood transfusion every week or two.

The good news is that in most cases, iron supplementation and a return to normal or even near normal hemoglobin levels will greatly improve one's energy, mood, and quality of life. People with mild to moderate anemia may also find that their bodies adjust over time to a bit less oxygen, just as those of people who live at high altitudes do. Some people whose anemia caused severe fatigue in the past will feel much less fatigued years later even if their hemoglobin level is unchanged.

What's Next?

As described in chapter 1, HHT involves more than nosebleeds and GI bleeding. AVMs can occur in the lungs, brain, liver, or spine, causing such medical complications as stroke, brain abscess, neurological problems, liver failure, and heart failure. Chapter 3 is all about AVMs—what they are and how they cause trouble, what screening tests are needed to find them, and how they can be treated to keep you healthy.

Chapter 3

HHT's Hidden Dangers
All about AVMs

Arteriovenous Malformations: Super-Sized Telangiectasias

Although nosebleeds are the most recognized symptom of HHT, they are just the tip of the iceberg. Most of HHT's serious health consequences are caused by *arteriovenous malformations*, or *AVMs*, which are much larger versions of telangiectasias. An AVM is an abnormal, direct connection between a vein and an artery in which capillaries are missing or deformed, but the veins and arteries that form an AVM are larger than those involved in telangiectasias. As noted earlier, the term *AVM* is typically used in medical literature to describe this type of direct connection occurring in the internal organs, regardless of absolute size, whereas *telangiectasia* is used for the same abnormality when it is on the skin or in mucous membranes (nose, mouth, GI tract).

AVMs are invisible from the outside and usually asymptomatic until a serious complication occurs. About 40 percent of people with HHT have AVMs in their lungs; approximately 5–20 percent have them in the brain; and about 1 percent have an AVM in the spine. While AVMs in the liver are actually the most common (found in about 75 percent of people with HHT), liver AVMs rarely cause symptoms or require any intervention.

Some of the most common serious complications from HHT result from lung and brain AVMs, so we'll talk about them first.[1]

Disaster Prevention: Finding and Treating Lung AVMs*

How Do Lung AVMs Cause Trouble?

Lung AVMs cause several serious problems. First, blood flowing through an AVM in the lung is not filtered effectively because the capillaries are

* Lung AVMs are sometimes called *pulmonary AVMs* or *PAVMs* in the medical literature.

missing. This means that bacteria, air bubbles, or blood clots traveling to the lungs through the bloodstream, which would normally be filtered or caught by the capillary bed (think of a fishnet or cheesecloth), can get through the AVM and travel back to the brain. If bacteria get lodged in a blood vessel in the brain, they can cause an *abscess* (infection), which can be life threatening. If a small clot or air bubble gets stuck in a blood vessel in the brain, it can cause an *ischemic stroke*, that is, a stroke caused by interrupted blood flow and lack of oxygen to part of the brain. Second, lung AVMs can hemorrhage (bleed) without warning, a serious and sometimes fatal event. Third, one or a few very large AVMs (or multiple tiny AVMs scattered throughout the lungs) can limit the lungs' ability to refresh the oxygen in the blood, so less oxygen reaches the brain and body, resulting in fatigue, shortness of breath, and the need for supplemental oxygen.

Most lung AVMs have *no symptoms* and give *no warning signs*. Therefore, *if you have—or suspect that you have—HHT, it's essential to be screened for AVMs in the lungs.* (Conversely, if someone has an AVM in the lungs, there's reason to suspect a diagnosis of HHT. About 85 percent of all lung AVMs occur in people with HHT.) Lung AVMs can be very small when first detected, but may grow larger during one's lifetime, particularly during adolescence. While doctors used to think that all lung AVMs were present from birth, there is now some evidence that lung AVMs can develop later. Lung AVMs tend to grow more rapidly during pregnancy, and a woman with *untreated* lung AVMs has a higher risk of hemorrhage from an AVM while she's pregnant. This is a good reason for women who have—or might have— HHT to get screened and treated for lung AVMs *before* becoming pregnant.

Adults and children have somewhat different risks from lung AVMs and their responses to treatment vary.

Screening Adults for Lung AVMs

The first test recommended for finding lung AVMs in adults is a *contrast echocardiogram*, also called an *echo bubble test* or a *bubble echo test*. In this test, saline (salt) solution is shaken up in a syringe, causing many tiny bubbles to form, then injected into a vein (this is the only part of the test that may cause mild discomfort), while a totally painless *ultrasound* (high-frequency sound) examination is performed to see whether the bubbles pass from the right side of the heart into the left side. Normally, the bubbles are trapped by capillaries in the lungs and do *not* get into the left side of the heart. But when there is a lung AVM, the normal capillaries are missing and filtering does not take place; instead, blood flows directly from an artery in the lung to a vein in the lung and then into the left side of the heart. This type of blood flow, which is abnormal, is called a *shunt* or *right-to-left shunt*. The blood containing the bubbles that are "shunted" into the left side of the heart is then pumped into the aorta, the large artery that carries oxygen-rich blood to the brain (and throughout your body). Since the test bubbles are very, very tiny, they are very unlikely to cause any problems in the brain. But if shunting exists, it means that other substances (such as blood clots, bacteria, or larger air bubbles) could get into the brain, potentially causing a stroke or abscess.*

Although the echo bubble test can't tell the exact number, location, or size of the AVM(s) in the lung, there is a grading system to measure about how many bubbles get through, or the severity of the shunt. The echo bubble test is very sensitive; even a very tiny AVM that is unlikely to cause any problems and is much too small to treat with current technology will allow some bubbles to get through the lungs. If the number of bubbles is very small, further testing of your lungs may not be needed. But if you have moderate or severe degree of shunting, you will need another test to determine the location and size of your lung AVM(s) in order to guide treatment decisions. This test is a *computed tomography (CT)* or *computerized axial tomography (CAT) scan*, which is a three-dimensional x-ray, sometimes with a special dye (*contrast* material) injected in a vein just before the test. Aside from the IV needle stick, this test is completely painless and takes only a few minutes to complete. It produces detailed images of your lungs, including the blood vessels.

Screening Children for Lung AVMs

Like adults, children in a family with an identified HHT gene mutation can have genetic testing with a blood test. If they *do not* have HHT, no further

---

* *Shunt* in this context refers to an abnormality in circulation. The word *shunt* may also be used to refer to abnormal openings or holes in the heart and elsewhere. These uses of the word refer to something completely different from the surgical shunt, which redirects the flow of fluid or blood to *correct* an abnormality, for example, in treating hydrocephalus.

screening is needed. But if they *do* have HHT, clinical testing is necessary to discover whether they have lung or brain AVMs. If no one in the family has had the genetic test but a parent has clinically diagnosed HHT, then *all* children in that family should have clinical testing for AVMs, whether or not they have nosebleeds or other symptoms.

There are some differences of opinion about what *types* of screening are necessary for young children who have no symptoms of lung AVMs. Many doctors believe that children up to 10–14 years of age who have no symptoms can be screened simply by monitoring their blood oxygen levels, using a test called *pulse oximetry*. This is done by putting a clothespin-like clip on the child's finger; the clip has special sensors and is attached to a machine that reads the level of oxygen (also called *oxygen saturation*) in the blood (fig. 3.1). This test, which takes a very short time, is not uncomfortable for the child and can be repeated as the child grows. But if a child's oxygen level is less than 97 percent, or if the child develops symptoms such as shortness of breath or difficulty keeping up in running or sports, then additional screening is necessary.

The screening recommended for younger children *who have symptoms* of a lung AVM and for all children older than about 10–14 years of age is the echo bubble test (the same test described above for adults). If the test shows

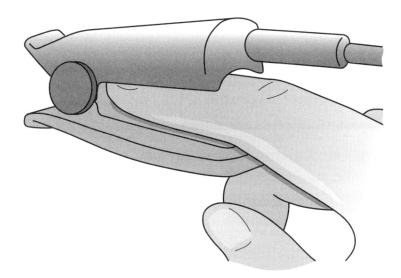

Figure 3.1 Pulse oximeter clipped onto index finger.

that the child has shunting, the doctor may recommend a CT scan of the lungs. Whether this step is recommended immediately or delayed until the child is older depends on the severity of shunting, the child's symptoms, and his or her medical history.

There are several reasons why doctors may try to minimize the use of CT scans in children. First, CT scans expose a child to radiation; if repeated numerous times, they can potentially increase the child's risk for cancer (although with the latest CT machines, the dose of radiation is very low). Additionally, research suggests that children with asymptomatic lung AVMs are less likely to have a stroke than adults with asymptomatic lung AVMs (though strokes do occur in some asymptomatic children), so earlier detection (and treatment) of lung AVMs may not be as important in children. Finally, children are more likely than adults to have a return of blood flow (*reperfusion*) to their lung AVMs after treatment with emboliza-tion (see below, "Treatment for Lung AVMs"), so the AVMs need to be retreated. Repeated embolization procedures also expose children to ra-diation, and unlike adults, children may need general anesthesia during the procedure. All things considered, it may be best to delay treatment of small to moderate-size lung AVMs in a young child who does not have symptoms, in which case it makes sense to delay the CT scan as well.

For older children or teenagers, an echo bubble test that shows moder-ate to severe shunting will usually be followed by a CT scan of the lungs to determine whether treatment is necessary.

Taking Care of Lung AVMs: Monitoring and Treatment

Once you and your children have been screened for lung AVMs, you're done for a while. If you have HHT but an initial screening does not reveal a lung AVM, you may still need some degree of monitoring to make sure that a lung AVM does not develop. And if you do have a lung AVM, follow-up tests are needed at various intervals throughout life to monitor AVM growth and/or whether treatments have been successful.

Monitoring Lung AVMs in Adults

Most doctors recommend periodic monitoring for people whose initial screening shows lung AVMs that are too small to treat. In adults, even when the first echo bubble test is negative (shows no shunting) the test should be repeated in about 10–15 years, because there is a small chance of developing a larger AVM that may require treatment. Some HHT Centers of Excellence base their recommendations for monitoring (with repeat testing) on a research study that used the shunt severity grading system to compare the degree of shunting on an echo bubble test with the size of AVMs found on CT scans done at the same time. The study showed that in people whose echo bubble test showed *no* shunting or *mild* shunting, the CT scan was very unlikely to show AVMs large enough to be treated. So for someone with only *mild* shunting, these centers recommend repeating the echo bubble test every five years and *not* doing a CT scan. Some doctors favor limiting the use of CT scans except in cases where it will provide uniquely valuable information. But other doctors prefer to use CT scans to further examine people who have mild shunting, because the grading system may be somewhat subjective and imprecise. New CT scanners use very low doses of radiation, and risks are minimal. Almost all doctors recommend a CT scan to examine the size and position of AVMs in people who show *moderate* or *severe* shunting on the first echo bubble test, since their AVMs are more likely large enough to need treatments. After treatment for a lung AVM, monitoring is done with a repeat CT scan about every five years to make sure that the AVM has been effectively eliminated.

Monitoring Lung AVMs in Children

Blood vessels grow more rapidly in children and adolescents than in adults, so more frequent monitoring (rescreening) is recommended. Children should have regular checkups to see whether any symptoms, such as shortness of breath, have developed. Monitoring lung AVMs may vary depending on where the child is cared for and on an assessment of his or her needs by the HHT team. HHT Centers of Excellence that rely on pulse oximetry for initial screening for lung AVMs in children *without* symptoms generally repeat the pulse oximetry to monitor changes in children over time, up to about 10–14 years of age. They would recommend an echo bubble test only if the child develops symptoms or after the child is 10–14 years old. Centers that prefer the echo bubble test as an initial screen for lung AVMs, even in babies and young children, may recommend repeating the test periodically to look for changes in the degree of shunting. In older children, recommendations for monitoring will depend on the degree of shunting (if any) seen on their first echo bubble test (as with adults).

Older children or teens require monitoring after treatment for a lung AVM. Some doctors lean toward using the echo bubble test, rather than a CT scan, to minimize radiation exposure. But as with initial screening for lung AVMs, some doctors prefer to use low-dose CT scans to monitor AVMs after treatment, because the echo bubble test may be difficult to grade. Depending on the child's individual circumstances, a follow-up CT scan about every five years after treatment may be recommended; this is something you should discuss with your child's HHT doctor after the procedure to treat his or her lung AVM.

Treatment for Lung AVMs

Whether your lung AVMs are symptomatic and whether they can be treated successfully depends in part on their size and number. Most small lung AVMs have no symptoms, and many people are unaware that they have one. But if you have one very large lung AVM or a number of moderate to large AVMs, the shunting of blood can decrease the amount of oxygen that gets into your blood, causing symptoms like shortness of breath, difficulty exercising, fingers turning blue, headaches, or dizziness. Similar symptoms can occur in people who have many very tiny AVMs spread throughout the lungs. Moderate and large AVMs can be treated to reduce these symptoms and prevent stroke and brain abscess. But multiple tiny AVMs throughout the lungs cannot be treated with currently available procedures (eventually, there may be a medication that reduces these AVMs). People with this pattern of AVMs can benefit from oxygen supplementation to help them walk and perform everyday physical activities.

The best way to eliminate the risks of a stroke or brain abscess due to a lung AVM is to get rid of the AVM. Before the development of noninvasive procedures for treating lung AVMs, people often had surgery to cut out the portion of the lung that contained the AVM. This surgery was risky and painful, and although it got rid of the AVM, it destroyed some of the healthy lung tissue as well. Fortunately, this surgery is no longer necessary. Now the most common treatment for lung AVMs is *embolization*, which plugs or seals up the blood vessel that supplies blood to the AVM. Ideally, embolization is performed *before* any serious complications occur (in adults and older children or adolescents), but many lung AVMs can be treated with embolization even *after* they have hemorrhaged, which prevents them from bleeding in the future.

Embolization is a virtually painless procedure done with x-ray-guided *angiography* (taking pictures of blood vessels), which in almost all cases requires no general anesthesia, no cutting, and no stitches. The procedure is usually done by an interventional radiologist, a doctor who specializes in the use of x-ray technologies to guide treatment procedures. The embolization is done in a special radiology suite (similar to an operating room) in the hospital, most often as an outpatient procedure. Recovery time is very short; you can resume normal activities after perhaps one or two days of rest.

In an embolization, a *catheter* (small tube) is inserted through a tiny incision into a large vein in your leg, then passed up into the arteries of the lungs. (Your leg is first numbed with local anesthesia, and you're given IV medication to relax.) A special dye or contrast is used during the procedure so that the blood vessels can be seen by x-ray. Sometimes this exploration of the blood vessels is done before actually treating the AVM, in which case it's called *pulmonary angiography*, but often this is done in one "session" along with the treatment procedure. Once the doctor knows exactly where and how the AVM is situated in the lungs, he or she can proceed with embolization.

Guided by x-ray, the doctor threads tiny steel coils or plugs through the catheter and inserts them into the artery leading to the AVM. If coils are used, they are tightly packed into the artery; plugs expand inside the artery, sealing off the blood flow. This treats the AVM by preventing blood from flowing into it. When treatment is successful, the tangled vessels of the AVM "die," and the shunt is eliminated (fig. 3.2). Blood is "rerouted" through other, normal vessels, and it can flow through capillaries, where debris is filtered out and oxygen is added in.

While embolization is not routinely used for young children who are asymptomatic, the procedure *is* used in young children whose lung AVMs cause symptoms like low oxygen levels in the blood, fatigue, and difficulty participating in active play. In symptomatic children, embolization can dramatically restore energy and health by raising oxygen levels in the blood.

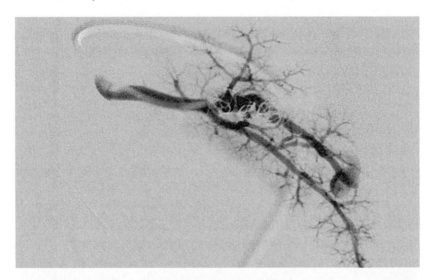

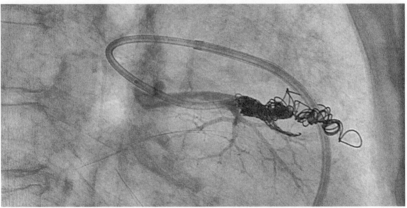

Figure 3.2 X-rays of lung AVM before and after embolization. *Top,* x-ray showing blood flow to the AVM through coils from a previous procedure; *bottom,* x-ray showing blood flow to the AVM completely blocked by embolization with a microvascular plug. Images courtesy of Dr. Sally Mitchell.

The waiting room in the ER was packed. My little girl was lethargic and weak. I held her for hours until we were finally called. Once the nurse hooked up the pulse-oximeter to her finger, it read 74 percent. I'll never forget seeing that number. The doctor said she had a large pulmonary arteriovenous malformation, causing her oxygen to be dangerously low. She was scheduled for an embolization. After the procedure, for the first time I noticed her lips were pink. I had always thought that grayish-blue color was just her. That's how she had always been. The next day, she got to come home, and it was so nice to see how much more energy she had. We always thought she was just a quiet girl. But she changed! And it was good.   —Connie

Embolization sometimes has to be repeated when blood flows back into the AVM despite the presence of coils or a plug. In rare cases, surgery may be necessary when *hemoptysis* (coughing up blood from the lungs) occurs after an embolization.

An Ounce of Prevention: Reducing Your Risk for Complications of Lung AVMs

If you have a lung AVM, whether it's been treated or not, there are several measures you can take to reduce the risk of medical complications.

Take antibiotics to prevent brain abscess. If you had an echo bubble test that showed any degree of shunting, or if you know you have a lung AVM (even if it's been treated), or if you haven't been screened yet and might have a lung AVM, there is one simple thing you can do to reduce the risk of getting a brain abscess due to bacteria going through the AVM and into your brain: take antibiotics when you have dental work or any other medical procedure that could introduce bacteria into your blood (for example, any type of endoscopy or surgery). This recommendation applies to children and adults.

Maybe you've heard that the American Heart Association no longer recommends prophylactic antibiotics for people with structural abnormalities of the heart (who are considered to be at risk for *endocarditis*, an infection around the heart). Your doctor might be confused by these recommendations and think they apply to people with HHT and lung AVMs. But this is not the case. Research has shown that people with untreated lung AVMs have a *much higher risk* of developing a brain abscess than people with structural heart abnormalities. In a study of 210 people with lung AVMs (excluding people whose lung AVMs were diagnosed because of a brain abscess), about 9 percent developed a brain abscess between the ages of 9 and 70. This is a relatively high risk for a very dangerous complication that can easily be prevented with a low-risk treatment with antibiotics.

Your doctor or dentist can prescribe oral antibiotics to take whenever you have a routine dental cleaning and to keep on hand in case you have a dental emergency. Taking one dose of the pills an hour before dental work is all it takes to lower your risk of having a brain abscess. Most people take penicillin, but if you are allergic to penicillin, you can take an alternative antibiotic such as clindamycin. If you must have surgery or another medical procedure, you can usually receive antibiotics through your IV rather than taking the pills.

Use an IV filter to prevent a stroke. Another prevention strategy recommended for people with lung AVMs is to use an IV filter when you receive any intravenous medication. The purpose of the filter is to prevent large air bubbles from getting into the IV line and possibly traveling to the brain, where they could cause a stroke. Air bubbles can sometimes cause a *transient ischemic attack (TIA)*, which results in temporary (transient) strokelike symptoms without any permanent impairment. You should request a filter whenever you must have an IV for a procedure. A 0.22-micron air filter is the best, but a standard blood filter, about 260 microns, is also effective in blocking larger bubbles. The air filter should be flushed before attaching it to the IV. Although filters cannot be used for injecting the IV contrast used for MRI or CT scans, you can request that extra care be taken to avoid any air bubbles in the syringe.

No scuba diving. Lung AVMs increase your likelihood of getting *decompression sickness (the bends)* when scuba diving. This condition can be very severe, affecting your lungs, muscles, nervous system, and other organs. Doctors recommend that anyone with lung AVMs, even after treatment, should not scuba dive. (Snorkeling is OK.)

When It's All in Your Head: Finding and Treating Brain AVMs*

The first time I heard of HHT was when my baby boy had a stroke.
—*Mike*

I always knew I had HHT, but I never understood what it meant, other than nosebleeds. It wasn't until my daughter had a bleed from a

---

* Brain AVMs are sometimes called BAVMs for short, or they may be called *cerebral* AVMs or *CAVMs*.

brain AVM—she was about 4 months old—that I went through screening for lung and brain AVMs; come to find out, I had one in my brain that had to be treated.   —*Leslie*

Between 5 percent and 20 percent of people with HHT have a brain AVM. These AVMs usually cause no symptoms and rarely cause any trouble, but when they do, the result can be devastating. The main complication of a brain AVM is *bleeding in the brain*, also called *intracranial hemorrhage (ICH)* or *hemorrhagic stroke*. Based on research to date, the risk of bleeding from an HHT-related brain AVM is about 1 percent per year. This means that in a given year, 1 out of every 100 people with a brain AVM may have a bleed. (This is actually lower than the risk for people with non-HHT or sporadic brain AVMs, whose risk of a bleed is about 2–4 percent per year.) In some cases, a brain AVM causes mild symptoms, such as headaches or dizziness, or more serious ones, such as seizures, that lead to its detection *before* it bleeds. But unfortunately, most people have no warning signs of a brain AVM until it causes a stroke.

When a brain AVM bleeds, it causes some degree of damage to the brain. Depending on the location and extent of bleeding, it may cause minor or temporary disruption in brain function; moderate to serious brain damage; or even death. Depending on the severity, there may be complete or almost complete recovery from a bleed in the brain, or only partial recovery; some people have permanent physical or cognitive disability after a brain hemorrhage. Children are likely to make a better recovery than adults, because their growing brains are more "flexible," or *plastic*, than those of adults: they form new nerve connections more rapidly, and one part of their brain can more readily take over the functions of another part.

Screening Adults for Brain AVMs

The only way to know for sure whether you have an AVM in the brain is to have an MRI scan. All North American HHT Centers of Excellence recommend this test for adults with known or suspected HHT.

It's very rare for a new brain AVM to develop in adulthood; so if you are diagnosed with HHT as an adult, you only need one MRI to test for a brain AVM. If the MRI scan shows that you do not have a brain AVM, then no further MRIs are needed. If the MRI scan shows that you do have a brain

AVM, your doctor will discuss treatment options with you. While the course of treatment may not always be clear, it's very important to know that the AVM is there. This knowledge can lead to faster and more effective treatment in the event of a bleed. Regular follow-ups (which may include physical exams and repeated MRIs) can help your doctor decide whether, when, and how to treat the AVM in the future.

The MRI scan uses a magnetic field and pulses of radio wave energy to make pictures of the brain; it is particularly useful for detecting blood vessel problems like AVMs. This test should be done both with and without *gadolinium* dye, a contrast material that makes the blood vessels more visible. Both can be done during the same appointment; first the test is done without the dye, then (as in the CT scan) the dye is injected into a vein through an IV line and the test is repeated.

During the MRI test, you lie down on a table that slides into a tubelike structure that is part of a special machine containing a strong magnet. While the pictures are being taken, the machine makes loud banging noises; usually, headphones with music are offered to block some of the noise. Some people feel claustrophobic in the enclosed tube of the machine. Those who are very anxious can be given a mild sedative to help them relax during the test. Use of an eye mask may also be helpful. But most people are comfortable in the MRI scanning machine. The MRI scan does not use radiation, and it is completely painless. The scan creates digital images that can be saved on a computer, viewed remotely, and copied onto a compact disc for you to keep with your medical records or share with another doctor or hospital. Note that *people who have certain types of metal (from injury or surgery) in their eyes or body should not have an MRI.* If you have had any metal implants or shrapnel injuries or have been a welder, ask your doctor whether it is safe for you to have an MRI.

Screening Children for Brain AVMs

Most doctors agree that *all* children with possible or definite HHT, whether or not they have symptoms, should have an MRI scan of the brain, both with and without contrast, to find out whether they have a brain AVM. This should be done during the first year of life, or whenever HHT is diagnosed in the child or his parent. Doctors do not know exactly when brain AVMs develop, but they are very rarely present at birth. In people with HHT who have brain AVMs, they are most likely to develop during the first few years of life, up until puberty. Because children can develop brain AVMs throughout childhood and adolescence, children whose first MRI scan does not reveal a brain AVM will need to have repeated testing (unlike adults). MRI testing should be repeated every five years until age 21 and then once more after that.

MRI testing for children, as for adults, is painless and does not expose them to radiation. Since babies and young children are not able to stay still during the test (which is essential for obtaining good pictures), they have to be sedated or anesthetized. But complications related to sedation are extremely rare in facilities that specialize in doing MRIs on children. Having your child's MRI done in a hospital or facility with experience in pediatric testing helps to ensure good-quality MRI images and a safe test.

Because new research may influence recommendations on screening children for brain AVMs, you should discuss the risks and benefits of MRI screening, as well as what is best for *your child*, with your HHT doctor before making a decision on this matter.

To Treat or Not to Treat a Brain AVM

Diagnosing a brain AVM with an MRI scan is fairly easy; deciding what to do when you find one is much harder. Treatment decisions depend on a number of factors: the size of the AVM, its location in the brain, certain structural features of the AVM, whether it has already bled, and whether or not it is causing any symptoms. If a brain AVM bleeds either before or after it's discovered on an MRI scan, the chances of it bleeding again increase to about 6 percent in the following year. Many people who have a brain hemorrhage from an AVM require some type of treatment to reduce the chances that the same AVM will bleed again in the future.

Sometimes *catheter angiography* is needed to evaluate the features of the AVM and make the best treatment plan. This involves inserting a small plastic tube into an artery in the groin; the tube is fed into the blood vessels of the brain, and pictures are taken while contrast material flows through the AVM. In adults, this procedure is performed under mild sedation in a special hospital room called a *neuroangio suite*. In children, it is performed with general anesthesia. The doctors specializing in this procedure are called *neuroradiologists*.

Based on the specific features of the AVM shown on angiography, doctors try to estimate the chance that bleeding from a particular brain AVM would be likely to cause significant brain damage. In addition, doctors must balance the risks and the benefits of treating the AVM. While there are few data on the rate of complications from treating HHT-associated brain AVMs, we do know that the risks of having a neurological deficit (that is, some degree of cognitive or physical impairment or disability) after treatment for any type of brain AVM is about 1–3 percent. It is possible that in some people treatment could result in complications as bad as or even worse than those resulting from a spontaneous bleed of the AVM.

Decisions about whether to treat a particular brain AVM are not easy, and there is no one-size-fits-all treatment plan. Most medical centers bring together a team of physicians, including a neurologist, a neurosurgeon, an interventional neuroradiologist, and possibly others, to evaluate brain AVMs and make recommendations for treatment and/or monitoring.

When to Watch and Wait

When an AVM is large and/or in a location that is not easily accessible (deep in the brain) but is not causing any symptoms, the risk of treatment may outweigh the benefits, and the best course of action may be to watch and wait. If this course is chosen, a schedule of monitoring with repeat MRI scans and neurological exams will be recommended. The repeat scans will show whether the AVM is growing, and the neurological exams will determine whether anything has changed in the patient's function. Of course, it is essential to report any new symptoms to your doctor immediately. Symptoms might include headaches, changes in vision, weakness, or changes in mental abilities such as difficulty remembering or concentrating. Brain AVMs can also cause seizures.

When to Treat

Sometimes a brain AVM bleeds suddenly and significantly, causing a stroke. The blood clot that results from the bleed may put life-threatening pressure on the brain. When this happens, emergency surgery is needed to remove the blood clot; sometimes the AVM can be removed at the same time.

When a person with HHT has a brain AVM that has not bled, is relatively small (less than 3 cm), and is located in the superficial part of the brain (closer to the outside of the brain), treatment may be considered. In such cases, the risk of treatment is likely to be very low (lower than the lifetime risk of a bleed). There are several ways to treat a brain AVM, including surgery, gamma knife, and embolization.

Surgery. If surgery is chosen, it will be necessary to open the skull in order to remove the AVM. The risks of this surgery depend on the size of the AVM and the experience of the neurosurgeon. The advantage of surgery is that it can successfully remove AVMs in almost 100 percent of cases, so the person is protected from a future bleed immediately.

Less invasive methods such as radiosurgery (gamma knife) or embolization should also be considered and may be preferable in some situations.

Gamma knife. The gamma knife is not a knife at all. It is a type of precisely targeted radiation that destroys the AVM and does minimal damage to the healthy brain tissue surrounding the AVM. With the gamma knife, there is no need to open the skull, and general anesthesia is not necessary in adults. Gamma knife treatment does not work immediately; it takes about three to four years for the AVM to disappear. Yearly MRI scans are performed after treatment to check on the size reduction of the AVM, and catheter angiography is performed to confirm that the AVM has been completely eliminated. The rate of success in treating a brain AVM with radiosurgery is about 90 percent.

Embolization. The technique for embolization of a brain AVM is very similar to what was described earlier for treatment of lung AVMs, except that the catheter is threaded into the blood vessels of the brain. Typically, a special type of glue (rather than a plug or coils) is used to block the blood vessels making up the abnormal connection between arteries and veins, which is called the *nidus* of the brain AVM. In about 40 percent of cases, treatment with embolization can completely cure a small brain AVM (fig. 3.3).

Embolization does not usually eliminate larger brain AVMs, but it is often used as a first step to reduce the size of the AVM or the high blood flow through the AVM. This procedure makes it safer to do surgery to complete the treatment and also makes it more likely that gamma knife treatment will be successful. Decisions about the best treatment for any brain

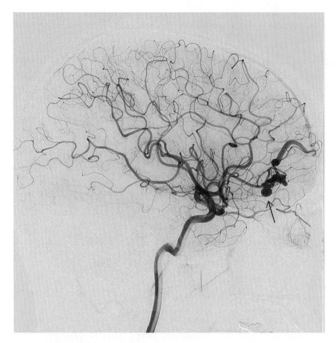

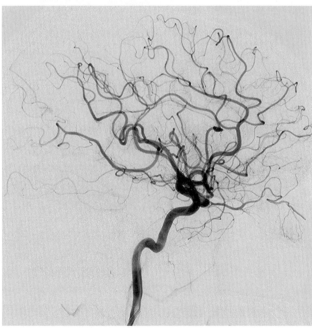

Figure 3.3 Brain AVM before and after embolization. *Top*, brain AVM appears as "blob" of vessels (see arrow); *bottom*, brain AVM eliminated following embolization with glue. Images courtesy of Dr. Karel terBrugge.

AVM must be made with input from a team of physicians and you, the patient (or parents of the patient).

First, Do No Harm: When to Treat Liver AVMs

No Screening for Liver AVMs

More than two-thirds of people with HHT have liver AVMs, but they rarely cause any symptoms or health problems. Most liver AVMs are low grade; that is, they do not interfere with the normal circulation of blood in the liver or with the functions the liver must perform to keep a person healthy. Doctors do not recommend screening for liver AVMs or treating liver AVMs when there are no symptoms. There is no good reason to treat liver AVMs preventively, because (a) they rarely become symptomatic and (b) intervention can make asymptomatic liver AVMs worse rather than better. In fact, embolization of liver AVMs has caused severe complications in several patients. Other procedures that can make a person with HHT and asymptomatic liver AVMs worse are liver biopsy (removing tissue from the liver with a small needle) and *endoscopic retrograde cholangiopancreatography (ERCP)*, a diagnostic procedure that involves putting a tube through the mouth and into the stomach, duodenum, and bile ducts. When it comes to liver involvement in HHT, it's good to think of that basic principle of medical ethics, first do no harm. If your doctor discovers liver AVMs incidentally, as a result of a medical test for another problem, or if you develop symptoms that could be a result of liver AVMs, you should not have any invasive tests or treatments before consulting an HHT Center of Excellence physician. Only a physician familiar with liver involvement and HHT can determine whether it's best to leave your liver alone or pursue invasive tests and treatment.

Treatment for Symptoms of Liver AVMs

Liver AVMs cause symptoms in about 5–8 percent of people with HHT. Symptoms almost always occur after age 50 and are two to three times more likely in women than in men. Unfortunately, when liver AVMs are symptomatic, they cause very serious health problems, including life-threatening bleeding, liver failure, and heart failure. Most treatments are aimed at reducing the *symptoms* caused by the liver AVMs. Unlike lung and brain AVMs, most liver AVMs cannot be treated safely with embolization.

> I've been very ill with HHT. My liver AVMs cannot be treated safely and my heart is failing. I am on so many medications to treat my heart, my anemia, and my nosebleeds, including regular iron infusions. I don't know if I am well enough to have a liver transplant—and if not, what will happen when all my medicines stop working?
>
> —*Alice*

Liver AVMs become symptomatic when they cause abnormal blood flow or shunting between major blood vessels in the liver. This can result in three main problems: high-output heart failure, portal hypertension, and biliary ischemia.

High-output heart failure is caused by liver AVMs that shunt a large volume of blood from major vessels in the liver back to the heart; the blood moves rapidly because the network of small blood vessels that would normally slow it down is missing. The heart must work harder to pump the high volume of blood, and eventually the heart loses efficiency. Some symptoms of high-output heart failure include shortness of breath, fatigue, swelling of the feet, and an enlarged heart. In mild cases, symptoms might only occur with strenuous exercise, while in severe cases, fatigue and shortness of breath occur with normal activities or even when resting. High-output heart failure can also cause *pulmonary hypertension* (increased pressure in the vessels of the lungs) in some people with HHT and liver AVMs.

Treatments for high-output heart failure include a low-salt diet, medications to reduce the amount of fluid retained in the body, iron supplements to control anemia (anemia worsens heart failure), and medications to correct irregular heart rhythms. IV infusions of bevacizumab (Avastin), a medication that slows the growth of new blood vessels, can be used to reduce symptoms of high-output heart failure by shrinking the liver AVMs and controlling bleeding. Usually these infusions must be repeated every year or two to keep symptoms under control.

Portal hypertension is an increase in blood pressure in the *portal vein*, one of the major blood vessels in the liver. This happens when the normal network of smaller blood vessels is missing, and a large volume of blood is shunted from the *hepatic (liver) artery* directly into the portal vein. Symptoms of portal hypertension can include swelling of the abdomen because of fluid collection (called *ascites*) and enlarged blood vessels in the esophagus (called *varices*) that are prone to bleeding. Hemorrhage from varices is a serious problem that can result in large, sometimes fatal blood loss. Symptomatic treatments for portal hypertension include blood pressure medicines and putting bands around varices to prevent bleeding.

Biliary ischemia is a lack of oxygen supply to the bile ducts, which carry bile from the liver to the gut. (Bile is a substance that helps in digestion, particularly in digesting fats.) Biliary ischemia happens when the blood supply to the bile ducts is reduced because of shunting through the liver AVMs. Without an adequate blood supply, the bile ducts are deprived of oxygen and the tissue is damaged. (This process is similar to an *ischemic* stroke, when part of the brain is deprived of oxygen because the blood supply is blocked by a clot.) Symptoms of biliary ischemia include abnormal liver blood tests, abdominal pain, and in severe cases jaundice (yellow skin and eyes) or infection of the bile ducts and fever. Treatments include pain medications and antibiotics for infection. Eating smaller, more frequent meals may help relieve symptoms.

Encephalopathy, or mental confusion, is another symptom of liver AVMs that may occur in combination with one of these three main problems. This happens when blood containing ammonia or other toxic substances normally processed by the liver is shunted between major veins in the liver and ends up going to the brain before being detoxified. These toxins cause confusion and disorientation that can usually be reversed with medications to lower the level of ammonia in the gut.

Other Treatments for Liver AVMs

One option sometimes considered for patients who don't respond to symptomatic treatments is *embolization* of liver AVMs. This procedure is technically similar to what was described above for treatment of lung and brain AVMs. But unlike embolization in the lung or brain, liver embolization is *very risky*, sometimes resulting in liver failure and death. It should be reserved only for life-threatening cases of heart failure caused by liver AVMs and should be performed only by a very experienced team of doctors.

A final option to consider when other treatments fail is a *liver transplant*. This major surgical procedure has significant risks for complications. It also involves lifelong maintenance on antirejection drugs. But for a small number of people, a liver transplant may be the only option for preventing death caused by heart failure from liver AVMs. Long-term survival is good for people with HHT who have a successful liver transplant; about 90 percent of them live five or more years after surgery.

Spinal AVMs

In addition to the lungs, brain, and liver, the spinal cord (the large bundle of nerves inside the spine) can be a site for AVMs. Spinal AVMS occur in about 1 percent of people with HHT. Because they appear so rarely, currently no routine screening is recommended for spinal AVMs.

Spinal AVMs can occur in children or adults. Diagnosis can be confirmed with an MRI scan. Like brain AVMs, spinal AVMs can bleed suddenly, resulting in arm or leg paralysis, or they may be discovered during medical evaluation for progressive neurological symptoms (such as gradually increasing weakness or numbness). These symptoms result from damage to nerves when the AVM presses on the spinal cord or on the spinal nerve roots, large nerves that branch from the spinal cord.

Depending on the size and location of the spinal AVM, symptoms can be mild or severe, ranging from back pain and odd sensations in the arms or legs to weakness or paralysis. Spinal AVMs are best treated with embolization using a gluelike substance to block blood flow in the AVM or with surgery. Treatment decisions are based on the location and size of the AVM, its symptoms, and whether or not it has bled. Embolization for a spinal AVM should be performed at a medical center with extensive experience treating this disorder.

Can Anything Else Go Wrong? Less Familiar Manifestations of HHT

Pulmonary Hypertension

I lost my independence with a diagnosis of pulmonary arterial hypertension (PAH) in its final stage. My health had so badly depleted by then, I was already grieving over the loss of what my life had been. I could no longer continue my career, my many charity work interests or even take my dog on the long walks we both enjoyed. It was six more years of ER visits, severe nosebleeds, fainting spells and undependable nosebleed treatments, before I received an additional diagnosis of HHT.   —Patti

Pulmonary hypertension (PH) is high blood pressure in the blood vessels of the lungs. Having PH does not mean that you have high blood pressure in all your blood vessels (*hypertension*); PH won't be detected by checking your blood pressure with a cuff on your arm. PH is a potentially serious condition that can contribute to disability or premature death.

About 11 percent of people with HHT have pulmonary hypertension. There are two types: The more common type is caused by high-output heart failure due to shunting of blood in the liver. This type of PH can also be caused by other factors (in people with or without HHT), such as severe anemia, irregular heart rhythms, leaky heart valves, or coronary artery blockages. The second type, which affects only about 1 percent of people with HHT, is *pulmonary arterial hypertension (PAH)*. PAH is caused by abnormal thickening of the walls of the blood vessels in the lungs, which narrows the vessels and results in a buildup of blood pressure in the lungs, heart failure, and inefficient blood flow to the body. PAH causes higher blood pressure in the lungs than PH and is more dangerous. PAH can occur in younger people with HHT, whereas PH is the result of a chronic process and occurs in adults.

The usual symptoms of PH are shortness of breath, fatigue, and other conditions associated with high-output heart failure. PAH also causes these symptoms and, as in Patti's case, can cause *syncope* (fainting, passing out) and chest pain, as the body is deprived of oxygen due to poor blood flow.

Screening for Pulmonary Hypertension

PH can be present before symptoms occur, and *screening for PH is recommended for all people with HHT*. Screening is done with an echocardiogram, which can be done at the same time as the echo bubble test for lung AVMs. The echocardiogram gives an *estimate* of pressures in the heart and lungs. If pressures are thought to be high, *cardiac catheterization* (a procedure similar to the one used for embolization of lung AVMs, in which a catheter is passed through a blood vessel in the leg) may be necessary to help diagnose the cause of PH by actually measuring blood flow and blood pressure in the heart and in the lung arteries. This is important in guiding treatment decisions.

Treatment for Pulmonary Hypertension

Treatment for PH includes managing the symptoms of high-output heart failure, as described for people with liver AVMs. For PAH, there are a variety of medication options to help reduce symptoms and extend life.

Lung AVMs present a difficult treatment problem in people who also have PH or PAH. Because of increased blood pressure in the lungs, AVMs are more likely to rupture (bleed). But treatment with embolization can also cause an increase in blood pressure in the lungs. For this reason, evaluation by a team of experts in HHT that includes a pulmonologist, preferably at an HHT Center of Excellence, is recommended for people with HHT who have pulmonary hypertension *and* AVMs in the lungs.

Juvenile Polyposis

My daughter Nicole was 11 years old when she started feeling sluggish and tired, often telling me, "I just don't feel good." When she was too tired to participate in her school's Field Day, I brought her to the doctor and he tested her for anemia. Her blood count was so low she was admitted to the hospital and received a blood transfusion the next day. Doctors did a colonoscopy to look for the source of her bleeding and her colon was "loaded with polyps." When the doctors learned that one side of our family had a history of colon disease and a lot of them had nosebleeds, they thought about *SMAD4*. They did genetic testing and Nicole was diagnosed with HHT and juvenile polyposis.   —*Robin*

You might recall our discussion earlier of the various genes that cause HHT. One of these, *SMAD4*, is the gene that causes HHT in 2–3 percent of cases. *SMAD4* also causes a genetic disorder called *juvenile polyposis*. In juvenile polyposis, numerous polyps develop in the colon and upper GI tract. (The word *juvenile* refers to the type of polyps, not to the age of the person who has the disease, which can cause symptoms in both childhood and adulthood.) People with this disorder have a high risk for developing cancer of the GI tract, so careful monitoring is necessary.

Symptoms of juvenile polyposis include bleeding from the rectum, blood in the stool, diarrhea, constipation, abdominal cramping or pain, chronic weight loss, and anemia. People with HHT and juvenile polyposis need expert care for *both* diseases and for management of interactions between symptoms of the two conditions (for example, GI bleeding from both polyps and telangiectasias). Surgery is often necessary to remove the polyps.

> Following her diagnosis, Nicole had a series of surgeries to remove polyps from her colon. She was also screened and treated for AVMs at an HHT Center of Excellence.   *—Robin*

A full discussion of juvenile polyposis is beyond the scope of this book. You can find more information from the National Institutes of Health, the Hereditary Colon Cancer Foundation (see the "Resources" section of this book), and your own health care providers.

Staying Up to Date

This book describes the current state of the art in HHT screening and treatment. But screening methods and treatment recommendations for HHT will continue to evolve as more is discovered about the genetics and the mechanisms behind HHT's many symptoms and research is done to evaluate the effectiveness of various medications for HHT.

To make sure that you get the best possible care for yourself and your family, it's essential to be informed about the latest research and clinical findings in HHT. The easiest way to do this is through Cure HHT's website, which regularly summarizes new developments in HHT care. Attending webinars and patient conferences will give you a deeper understanding and a chance to direct your questions to scientists and doctors involved with HHT research and treatment. If possible, seek your care at an HHT Center of Excellence; these centers are likely to offer the most current treatment techniques and procedures. You can also search the Internet for articles in scientific journals (a librarian can help you if you're not sure where to look). It may be difficult to decode the scientific jargon in some of these articles, but if something strikes you as intriguing, you can take it to your doctor or

HHT Center of Excellence and ask whether the findings have any relevance for your treatment.

How about Some Good News?

In the first three chapters, we've discussed so many possible complications of HHT that you might feel a bit overwhelmed. But let's keep a few things in mind: (1) not everyone has all (or even any) of these complications; (2) for every complication, there are treatments that can make it more manageable; (3) there are several measures that you can take to *prevent* complications; and (4) the most serious complications of HHT usually occur later in life, at a time when you may have completed your career and raised your family.

HHT is a chronic disease for which there is as yet no cure. But in general, if you know you have HHT, you can manage your symptoms with preventive measures and regular medical care. Your HHT may require lifelong maintenance, but you can still have a full life, going to school, working, seeing your friends, finding a romantic partner, parenting, enjoying leisure activities, and pursuing your interests and passions. In spite of having nosebleeds, anemia, or pulmonary AVMs, most people with HHT can live satisfying and happy lives.

> Neither I nor anyone else in my extended family thinks of HHT as the thing that defines us. We're an energetic, active, physically fit, even athletic bunch. As a group, we're healthy most of the time. Dealing with our HHT is not what we do in life—we've got a lot more interesting stuff going on!
>
> —*Ernie*

Of course, as we've seen, some people develop serious health problems or disabilities because of HHT. But it's possible to adapt to changes in your physical abilities and find different ways to participate in activities you enjoy—or discover new activities that fit your energy level and lifestyle. And it's possible to find meaning in life, to feel loved, and to value yourself even when it's hard to get through the day. In an article on the Pulmonary Hypertension Association website, a woman with HHT and PH put it this way:

I'm still learning to accept my "bad days" and enjoy my "good days." Bad days are when I can't muster the energy to get out of bed and go to work . . . when I have the opportunity to babysit my nieces and nephews and have to decline because I just do not have the energy. Good days are when I feel like my "old" self. I can do normal, simple things like grocery shopping, house cleaning and putting in a good day of work without exhausting myself. With the love of my family, all my days are truly blessed.[2]

Part II provides a menu of tools you can use to have the best life possible with HHT. In the next three chapters, we'll look at strategies to manage the impact of HHT on your health, your emotions, and your daily life; how you can cope with the effects of HHT on your family relationships, communicate more effectively with your family about HHT, prepare for parenting, and teach your children about HHT; and how you can advocate for better insurance coverage and medical care, legislative support, public awareness, and funds for HHT.

Part II

Living Well with HHT

Chapter 4

Taking Care of Yourself
HHT and Your Emotional Health

You are not crazy, but what you are going through *physically* is not normal, no matter how many doctors try to tell you it is.　　—*Joy*

HHT invades our families, interrupts our daily lives, and intrudes on our work and leisure. Several characteristics make HHT particularly hard to manage. Like many chronic illnesses, HHT is a lifelong condition with no cure (yet). Its symptoms wax and wane, and it has an unpredictable course. Serious problems can occur at any time—or never. Nosebleeds can be under control for a few years and then return with a vengeance. Youth and middle age may be uneventful, and then GI bleeding or liver involvement takes the shine off your "golden years." HHT can also interact dangerously with other illnesses that anyone may develop, such as cancer or heart disease.

The combined physical, emotional, and social effects of HHT influence how we feel about life in general. To a large extent, the severity of medical symptoms or complications determines our quality of life with HHT, but personalities and social factors also influence how strongly HHT affects our overall happiness. These factors include family and social support; coping skills; other medical or social stresses; positive or negative attitudes and beliefs about illness; and access to medical care, rehabilitation, education, and other resources. Some of these factors, such as having other medical problems, are beyond your control. But you *can* take control of other factors, for example, increasing your network of social supports, better educating yourself about HHT, and using various coping strategies to effectively deal with stress.

You can't eliminate HHT, but you can learn to limit its negative effects on your physical and mental health. This means practicing the preventive measures outlined earlier in this book, getting treatment when it's required, and making changes to improve your quality of life with HHT. It's important to note that after a period of adjustment and learning to manage their symptoms, many people experience *positive* feelings in response to HHT, such as self-acceptance, pride, confidence, and greater appreciation for life.

But even with the best attitude, support, and circumstances, HHT is likely to cause predictable increases in stress when symptoms become severe or affect work or family life. In this chapter, we'll look at some "stress points" for people with HHT and ways to manage them. First we'll look at strategies for coping with the more serious *physical* manifestations of HHT, such as energy limitations because of chronic fatigue, anemia, or heart failure and disabilities caused by stroke, brain hemorrhage, or brain abscess. Next, we'll discuss how to cope with normal, expectable *emotional* responses to HHT, as well as how to recognize when your emotional responses to HHT are beyond normal and you could benefit from help provided by a mental health professional.

Nosebleeds, because they are the most common and most frequent symptom of HHT, cause a great deal of emotional distress and have a negative impact on quality of life for many people with HHT. For this reason, nosebleeds, nosebleed treatment, and strategies for managing and coping with nosebleeds were discussed extensively in chapter 2. The current chapter focuses on the less common but often more serious or chronic manifestations of HHT and how to cope with them.

Coping with Physical Limitations Caused by HHT

One of my favorite sayings about unpredictable illnesses is, "Hope for the best, but plan for the worst." You might suppose that you can protect yourself from stress by not thinking about all the bad things that can happen to you because of HHT. But being prepared for a variety of possible symptoms or problems can actually help you manage your disease, ultimately reducing its stressful consequences. If you can imagine stressful events and mentally rehearse some ways to deal with them, you can cope better emotionally if or when these events occur.

Fatigue, Weakness, and Disability

Anemia, heart failure, pulmonary hypertension, low oxygen levels, and stroke or brain abscess may occur with HHT at any age. Anemia caused by severe GI bleeding and heart failure are more common in older people, and stroke is more likely in people who have untreated brain or lung AVMs. These conditions can cause fatigue, limit exercise tolerance, and make everyday activities difficult.

> My symptoms grew so bad. If I walked upstairs in my house, I got dizzy and short of breath. I had nosebleeds and sometimes fainted. I was hospitalized twice from being unable to breathe. At my daughter's wedding, I was barely able to move. I had to give my dog up for adoption because I couldn't walk him anymore. After working for the past 25 years, I went on disability; I was wearing an oxygen tube and needed a wheelchair to move more than a hundred feet!   —*Patti*

When you experience severe fatigue, you may have to give up certain things that you enjoyed doing in the past. It may be helpful to think about adjusting your goals to better fit your energy level. Try to *set priorities* and let go of activities that aren't as meaningful or critical to you. That way you will have more energy for the hobbies, chores, or social activities you regard as most important. For example, if you want to go to a theater performance or out to dinner at a friend's house, make that a priority and save your energy by not doing chores that day. On a bigger scale, think about what life goals are most important to you. Do you want to spend more time working? Seeing your grandchildren? Traveling? Enjoying time with your friends or your partner? If you focus on activities that are most fulfilling (or perhaps most important) to you and cut back on others, you will feel less limited than if you try to do everything and end up struggling all the time.

Whether you are limited by fatigue because of anemia or weakness owing to a stroke, try to *set goals that you know you can achieve*. If you're tired most of the time, set the bar low and don't expect much from yourself. When you accomplish something, reward yourself. You can always set the bar higher the next time.

> Thanks to new medicines, I am alive and stable. We moved out of our second floor townhouse to a condominium with elevators. I have

learned to manage my life around whether it is a good or bad health day. I am able to do some light housework, including cooking, which I love.

—*Patti*

Making some lifestyle changes can help you conserve your energy. If possible, *get help from others* for energy-intensive tasks such as housecleaning, grocery shopping, or raking the leaves. *Use technology to reduce energy expenditure.* For example, shop online instead of walking through the mall, or use an electric scooter or stair lift to get around more easily. *Get enough sleep every night.* Eight hours is a great goal, but you may need more. If your schedule allows, take a nap during the day. *Meet your nutritional needs.* Your doctor or a dietician can help you determine what's best for you. A healthful diet will help you function at your best.

Stroke survivors or people with severe weakness resulting from heart failure may need help with *activities of daily living (ADLs)* such as bathing, dressing, eating, using the bathroom, walking, paying bills, and driving. It's best to get this help from a number of different family members—or from paid helpers if you can afford them—to avoid putting too much stress on one person. *Rehabilitation services* such as physical, occupational, and speech therapy can help you increase your independence after a stroke, teach you how to conserve energy, improve your ability to function with chronic fatigue or weakness, and guide your family in providing the best kind of help for you.

If you don't have the energy or stamina to get out socially, try to *stay socially connected* in other ways. Social relationships and support are critical to your physical and mental well-being. Talk on the telephone, ask people to visit you at home, or stay in touch electronically by e-mail, Skype, and social media. These methods are especially helpful in keeping up with friends and family who live far away. Facebook hosts several HHT patient groups, providing an opportunity to meet other people who have HHT, share stories and health information, and find emotional support.

If you are dependent on blood transfusions or make frequent visits to the ER or hospital for other complications, you may feel that your entire life revolves around just trying to survive. If you're in this situation, try to find enjoyable ways to spend the downtime in the hospital, and plan *pleasurable experiences* during the times between hospital or doctor visits. Spending more time doing things you enjoy (even if you can't do *all* the things that you like) is good for your mood and boosts your motivation to continue taking care of your health.

> My mom had severe GI bleeding and went to the hospital twice a week—once to check her hemoglobin and once to get a blood transfusion. She made friends and joked around with the other patients and the nurses. She always brought a book to read or she called friends on her cell phone. On the way home, she and my dad would stop for lunch at their favorite restaurant. On days when she didn't need to go to the hospital, she had friends come over to visit, listened to music, organized photos, sent e-mails, or did other things that didn't take much energy but were fun and made her feel that she was more than her illness. —*Sharon*

Work Limitations and Disability Benefits
The Americans with Disabilities Act and Accommodations

People with HHT may have to reduce their work hours or retire early because of serious complications or limitations to their ability to do their jobs. More often, they may need changes to their work duties or hours (legally called *accommodations*) because of nosebleeds, reduced energy levels, weakness, or other problems that might affect their job performance. Many people prefer not to tell their employers that they have HHT, but if you need to take frequent or lengthy breaks because of nosebleeds, or if you need to do a less physically demanding job because of anemia, you may benefit from telling your employer and asking for accommodations so that you can continue to work as long as possible. The Americans with Disabilities Act (ADA), designed to protect people from discrimination on the basis of a disability or medical condition, includes the right to accommodations at work.

You can learn more about the ADA on the website www.ada.gov. If you work for a large company, there may be a staff person in the human resources department who can help you with disability issues. Changes in work schedules or hours are among the most frequent workplace accommodations made for people with disabilities. However, if you are not able to complete the basic functions of the job even with the accommodations, you may have to retire or find different work.

Disability Benefits

It is important to familiarize yourself with your employer's policy on sick leave and disability benefits, as well as the financial supports available if you need to take time off or leave your job because of health problems. Many large employers offer short- or long-term disability insurance; sometimes the employer pays for the insurance, and sometimes the employee can choose the insurance and pay for it voluntarily. If your employee benefits are inadequate or nonexistent, you might want to purchase private disability insurance or long-term-care insurance to provide an income in case you become disabled. You may be able to purchase disability insurance through a professional association, union, or guild without providing medical records. However, if you have HHT, it may be difficult to buy private disability insurance. Although the Affordable Care Act of 2010 prevented *health* insurers from excluding customers based on a preexisting condition, companies that sell *disability or life* insurance *are* allowed to exclude people who have an illness or condition that's likely to cause a disability.

Social Security Benefits

Whether or not you have private or employer disability benefits, you may be eligible for disability payments through Social Security Disability Insurance (SSDI) if you are no longer able to work. You will need to file an application, submit medical records, and perhaps be interviewed or examined by a doctor. Many people seek assistance from an attorney when applying for SSDI, but it is possible to apply on your own. For more information and to get an application, visit www.ssa.gov/disability. If you are granted SSDI, you will become eligible for health insurance under Medicare regardless of your age. You may be able to work part time and still qualify for SSDI, but there is a limit to how much money you can earn while receiving SSDI payments.

To be eligible for SSDI, you must have worked for a certain number of years and paid into the Social Security fund. Younger people or those who have not worked long enough to get SSDI may qualify for Supplemental Security Income (SSI), depending on their financial need. If you receive SSI, you may also be eligible for Medicaid (Medical Assistance). Consultation with a certified financial planner, insurance agent, or lawyer specializing in disability may help you identify your options for private and/or government disability benefits.

Coping with Emotional Consequences of HHT

You're (Probably) Not Crazy—It Just Feels That Way

> I went to my new doctor armed with my suspicions and articles about screening and general information on HHT. I believe the doctor truly thought I was a complete nut (or hypochondriac) as I showed him my research and taught him about this "rare" thing called HHT.
>
> —*Lorna*

> So many doctors called me a phony and a prima donna—until finally someone saw I was really sick and believed me.   —*Maria*

As described in chapter 1, HHT causes a wide range of symptoms that vary from person to person. Combined with a lack of public awareness and physician knowledge, this leads to delays in getting a proper diagnosis. If your experience resembles that of most people with HHT, there was a very long time between your first symptom and finding out that you had HHT. You may have started to feel a little crazy as you went from doctor to doctor with a variety of mysterious complaints that no one could explain.

And when you finally got a diagnosis and tried to tell your family about it, they may not have believed that HHT could have anything to do with them. Maybe they tried to persuade you that you were blowing things out of proportion. Even though you were trying to do them a favor, you may have felt discredited and questioned your own sanity. Or you may have felt sad, confused, or frustrated by physical limitations or disability, being unable to work or continue enjoyable hobbies because of your health, losing a parent to HHT, or having a child with complications from HHT. For all these reasons, you may wonder whether you're "losing it."

Although having HHT can feel like being on an emotional roller coaster, it does not cause any mental disorders. The genes for HHT are *not* associated with psychiatric or mental illness, and people with HHT are no more likely than anyone else to have a particular psychiatric disorder. But although you're not crazy, having HHT can be emotionally distressing. And most people find certain HHT-related events particularly stressful; these events include getting diagnosed, telling your family (or future spouse or partner) about HHT, having a child (or grandchild) with HHT, going to the hospital, becoming seriously ill, and experiencing the death or serious illness of a close family member. Some emotional upheaval in response to these events is normal, but most people "bounce back" after a period of adjustment. Let's look at coping techniques to manage normal emotional ups and downs and what to do when your emotions interfere with your ability to manage life.

Challenge Negative Thoughts

> My doctor came in and told me I had a pulmonary arteriovenous malformation in my lung. She told me it was extremely rare, and they would have to find a specialist to treat it. One of the nurses was so excited to learn about a new rare disorder. . . . To me it wasn't exciting—it was terrifying. I felt alone and scared.   —*Tanya*

It's common for people to feel scared when newly diagnosed with HHT, especially when the diagnosis is made because of a serious complication. This and other emotional reactions can happen so quickly that they seem to be involuntary, but often our emotions are tied to our thoughts; what we *think* about a situation has a lot to do with how we *feel* about and react to it. During times of stress, it's common to have irrational thoughts, and these thoughts can trigger negative emotions. One thing you can do to manage emotions like fear, anger, and sadness is examine your thoughts and look for alternatives to the thoughts that don't really make sense.

The following quote from an anonymous post on the Cure HHT website contains two thoughts presented as feelings:

> I am so tired of people telling me that it's not so bad or that it could be worse. And you know, they are right—it could be worse. But I feel like no one understands my point of view and that I am alone in this.

The writer probably means something like this: "I feel sad because I *think* no one understands me and I *think* that I am all alone." But the thought "No one understands me" is almost always an exaggeration of reality. While it may be true that not *everyone* understands your point of view, there is almost always *someone* who can empathize with your feelings. If we look more closely at the thought "I am alone in this," we can see that that's not true either. You and I—and most people with HHT—have at least one family member or friend to whom we can turn for comfort and support. And besides, there are more than a million people in the world with HHT, so how can any of us *really* be alone in this?

Examining the thoughts behind your feelings can help you change your emotional responses to stressful events. If you challenge negative thoughts, you might find that positive thoughts about your situation make just as much sense as negative ones. This will help you feel better not only right away but in the long run. For example, when you think to yourself, "I guess I'm not really alone, my sister (or best friend or partner) is always there for me," you are more likely to ask your family and friends for support. Or if you think, "I'm one of over a million people with HHT—that's a lot of people who know what I'm going through," you're more likely to connect with the HHT community on Facebook, at a conference, or on the phone. All these folks can share your experience and give you emotional support. And when you have more connections with other people, you will no longer feel so alone.

Other irrational negative thoughts that people may have when they are dealing with the stress points of diagnosis, increasing symptoms, or medical procedures include the following:

- I can't handle this.
- I'm being punished.
- There's no hope for me.
- I'll always feel awful.

It's easy to see how these thoughts can lead to feeling sad, angry, helpless, or hopeless. And yet, if you examine each of these thoughts rationally, you can see that they are not true. If you look objectively at each statement, you can probably find a way to contradict it with a more realistic thought. Below are some positive thoughts that can replace the negative ones above:

- *I've handled challenges before.* What's more, I know lots of other people who've handled serious illnesses. It might take some help, but I can do it.

- *I have an inherited disease.* It has no relationship to anything I've done or have not done, so it can't be a punishment.
- *There are lots of reasons for me to have hope.* There are many treatments that can help me. Research is under way to find better treatments for HHT. My life may have some limitations, but I can still enjoy many things.
- *Feelings come and go.* I've experienced anger and sadness before, and I've also experienced happiness and contentment. The feelings I have now will not last forever. I will feel good again.

Reframing: Tell Yourself a Different Story

One way to keep negative emotions under control and tap into your emotional strengths is to create a more positive narrative to describe your life experiences. In the process of telling a new story, you may discover or create a new way of understanding your reality that can lead to a stronger sense that your life has purpose, meaning, or value. By applying alternative (more positive) words or labels for yourself or your feelings and different (more positive) explanations for experiences that might seem terrible or overwhelming, you can alter your interpretation of events; this is called *reframing*. Even though you can't change the event itself, changing the story you tell yourself increases your ability to cope with (and maybe even benefit from) an experience that you expected to be harmful. Reframing helps you "make lemonade out of lemons," allowing you to find the benefits of living with HHT.

Having this positive label for myself as a "survivor" helps me to see the world in a "half-full" kind of way. If I was labeled as a "victim," I wouldn't be the person I am now and I wouldn't be as happy. The positive label of being a "survivor" had an enormous influence on me because it gave me the strength to keep going and progressing despite the numerous walls that I had to climb over. The value I have gained staying positive throughout situations that seemed unbearable and dismal, and the view I have of the world now, could not be learned anywhere else, and I wouldn't trade anything in the world for it. And because I had this positive label for myself, I was able to see life in the optimistic way I do now. I consider myself one of the luckiest men to roam the earth, and I always receive the same response: "Luckiest man? But that was such a terrible thing to go through." And I always reply with, "It's only terrible if you make it that way."   —*Aaron*

After a brain abscess and stroke due to HHT, Aaron's use of reframing led to feelings of happiness and empowerment. Aaron changed the label he used for himself (from "victim" to "survivor"), and he changed his interpretation (story) of his medical situation: rather than being "unbearable," it heightened his positive feelings of optimism and gratitude.

Mindy had a similar transformation. Focusing on how well she coped with HHT rather than on the problems it caused, she came to appreciate her own character strengths and to recognize her value as a role model for dealing with adversity.

Having HHT can be challenging, but I have found a bright side to it, as well. I am passing on a new inheritance to my children. Along with the dreaded HHT, they are receiving the lessons that perseverance, courage, and good self-care are precious commodities. They have watched me struggle and watched me heal. They have seen me learn to let myself be weak and reach out for support. They have heard my prayers for strength and seen me live my motto "never give up!" through good times and bad.   —*Mindy*

Reframing is also helpful for people dealing with chronic illness or disability related to HHT. As discussed earlier, severe fatigue, shortness of breath, and heart failure can lead to limited energy, difficulty with physical activities, and a loss of one's roles as worker, homemaker, and so forth. Sometimes these losses contribute to feelings of depression, low self-esteem, or hopelessness. But reframing can help you focus on what you *can* do rather than on what you *can't* and get more enjoyment from your hobbies and relationships.

I enjoy reading, knitting for fun, and social life with my friends. I have learned to enjoy my relaxed lifestyle after a hectic career with tight deadlines. I count my blessings and live happily one day at a time.   —*Patti*

Like Aaron, Patti was able to find the positive side (having a relaxed life-style) of a "negative" event (not being able to work), helping her to enjoy life in spite of restrictions imposed by her illness.

Make the Mind-Body-Relationship Connection

I have developed a very strong commitment to pursuing physical, emotional, relational, and spiritual health.   —*Mindy*

A commonly used model of health today is the *bio-psycho-social model*. According to this model, the interplay between physical, psychological, and social factors (body, mind, and relationships) determines our overall health and well-being. Improvements in any of these areas can have a positive effect on the others. Awareness of this mind-body-relationship connection is especially helpful in coping with HHT-related health issues. Even if you can't eliminate a particular physical symptom, you can harness the mind-body-relationship connection to reduce stress or pain by changing your thinking, emotions, or social interactions. Just as we can alter emotions by changing our thoughts, we can reshape our thoughts and emotions by engaging our bodies in movement and exercise. Likewise, we can improve physical health and recovery from illness through mental relaxation and supportive social relationships.

Exercise

When I'm stressed out, I take the kids to the park; we take a walk, go on the swings. We take ten minutes to be together and just breathe!   —*Joy*

Physical exercise or movement of any kind has a beneficial effect on your mood. It helps to reduce anxiety or the blues. Exercise releases endorphins, the brain chemicals associated with "runner's high," which create feelings of joy or contentment. Exercise builds stamina, balance, and strength, which can help you function better as you age or cope with illness. And exercise creates a more positive body image, which can override negative images associated with disability or waning strength and energy.

Some people with HHT are able to engage in challenging physical exercise like running, climbing, and cycling; others walk, play a little golf, or swim a few laps. All of these activities increase self-confidence while contributing to overall health and fitness. Gentle exercises such as chair yoga, water aerobics, or short walks, which may be possible for people with fatigue, weakness, or limited mobility, provide many of the same benefits. If you're not sure what type of exercise is best for you, ask your doctor to help you design a personalized exercise routine. Remember, even 10 minutes of exercise a day can boost your mood, strengthen your body, and enhance your sense of well-being.

Relaxation

How do I keep my sanity? I do yoga, read books, and work on puzzles.
—*Joy*

To relax in the hospital, I watch YouTube, draw, play games, and talk on the phone. —*Nicole*

Relaxation is a powerful tool for reducing mental stress, managing pain, and experiencing good feelings in your body. Most people use some form of relaxation to unwind from the normal stresses of everyday living. Some common examples include taking a hot bath, listening to music, hanging out with friends, or playing with a pet. All of these involve pleasurable sensations and engage our attention, taking our focus away from troubling thoughts, physical pain, or distressing emotions.

Mindfulness

In addition to the above-mentioned common stress reducers, many people use techniques designed to foster *mindfulness*, a deeper level of relaxation, awareness, and well-being. These techniques include exercises like *yoga* and *tai chi*, which combine slow movement, balance, deep breathing, and mental focus; *meditation*, which aims to calm or focus the mind, often using breathing techniques, chanting, or repetition of a soothing word; and *guided imagery*, which uses mental images (such as waves lapping the shore) to reduce tension, pain, or fear. These techniques can be learned at exercise studios, community centers, and adult education centers. Public libraries often carry books and CDs that can guide you through meditation or imagery. Some hospitals offer group mindfulness classes, and mental health professionals may use mindfulness techniques in individual therapy practices.

Social Support

Support from relationships with family, friends, and community is essential to mental health. People who have large networks of social relationships, as well as a few close emotional connections with loved ones, are generally better able to recover from illness, less likely to be depressed, and more likely to remain physically and mentally active into their senior years. Social support plays an important part in reducing the negative impact that HHT can have on a person's health and emotions.

It's especially helpful to have a friend or neighbor lined up to give you extra support at times when you're most likely to be stressed. If you have chronic symptoms of HHT or need frequent treatments, it's a good idea to identify several people with whom you can talk comfortably about your health issues and to whom you can turn when you need backup. You might find that some friends are better at giving you *emotional support* (having fun, hanging out, and talking), while others can be counted on for *practical support* (helping with household chores, acting as your advocate at medical appointments, or giving you a ride to the doctor or grocery store). You might also want to talk to a counselor or clergyperson or chat with other people on social media.

> You have to get into the community of illness; the more people you talk to, the more you learn. And you're not alone—you can join Cure HHT on Facebook and share that you have HHT. When I posted, three people contacted me. It's good to find one person to talk to you or hold your hand while you're getting test results.   —*Joy*

Remember that not all "close" relationships are supportive. When you are sick or emotionally taxed, it helps to spend time on the relationships you find reliably enjoyable, helpful, and supportive and put less energy into those that tend to be draining or cause distress. A degree of disagreement in close relationships is normal, but it's healthy to table those conflicts during times when one person in the relationship clearly needs more support. If the person you are turning to for help is not able to put grievances on the back burner, you may need to seek support from someone else.

Maintain Your Identity: You're Not *Just* HHT

People differ widely in the extent to which HHT shapes their identity. Some people look at HHT strictly as something they *have*, while others see it as something they *are*. In a recent study of life experiences with HHT, one young woman put it this way: "I'm not ashamed or embarrassed about it. . . . It's just a part of me and a part of my daily life."[1] Some people are proud of living well with HHT and discuss it openly with friends or publicly on social media, while others prefer to discuss HHT only with their family and doctors. There's no right way. But what's essential to good mental health is keeping HHT in its place, that is, not letting it become the only thing that defines you as a person. You are much more than an illness. You're an individual with interests, dreams, and accomplishments.

> I wouldn't say that my symptoms from HHT prevent me from living my life. . . . I don't let it keep me from trying to do the things I want to do. I am the only person that can stop me from becoming who I want to be. —*Gary*

After you've been evaluated and treated and learned preventive health practices to guard against complications, you probably don't want to spend every waking moment worrying about HHT. Unless you have severe complications from HHT, you can do most of the same things that anyone else can do, such as playing sports, traveling, having children, or changing careers. You can take some risks and reach for your goals.

> I've been treated for a lung AVM. I know when to get my next CT scan and I'm careful to take my antibiotics before going to the dentist. There's not much more to do about it right now. I get some pretty bad nosebleeds now and then, but I'm not going to stop doing the things I love because I *might* have a nosebleed. I've got my bucket list and I'm going to get the most out of life while I still can! —*Edward*

A goal to strive for is to keep the balance between dealing with your HHT and engaging fully in the rest of your life. Sometimes your health needs will tip the balance, and you may need to adjust your life goals or spend more of your day managing HHT health concerns. But remember that you're *still you* and can find meaning and enjoyment through a variety of roles, relationships, and activities that don't require physical strength.

Have the Last Laugh

> Years back, when my kids were little, we went to a Halloween party. I was dressed up as a witch with a black hat and green make-up. It was an exceptionally hot day, and I worried about getting a nosebleed. When I walked in, the hostess looked at me and said, "Wow, your witch blood is *so* realistic—where did you buy that?" And I just laughed out loud, because I knew it must have happened—a nosebleed was my "make-up" secret!
>
> —*Sharon*

Humor is a wonderful antidote to sadness and anxiety. Laughter helps reduce stress, lower blood pressure, and reset your attitude. It's another way to reframe a serious event by finding its funny flip side. Laughing at *yourself* is particularly therapeutic and has the added benefit of putting others at ease with your situation.

> I hike, kayak, and garden in my free time and have learned how to thrive even in the midst of struggles and pain. As Monty Python says, "I'm not dead yet!" Far from it—I am very much alive. I can tell from that little bit of blood that leaked out of my nose this morning.
>
> —*Mindy*

When to Get Help from a Mental Health Professional

Seeing a mental health professional can be beneficial even if you don't have a psychiatric disorder. Many people seek counseling or psychotherapy to help them cope with health setbacks, deal with grief after losing a loved one, or solve difficult problems in family relationships. Sometimes you just need more support than friends and family are able to give, especially when a stressful event affects everyone in the family.

But some people with HHT *do* experience psychiatric disorders. Although HHT does not *cause* mental health disorders, it does not *prevent* you from developing the same mental health disorders that anyone else can experience. Just as you can have HHT and develop unrelated medical problems like diabetes or cancer, you can have HHT and an unrelated psychiatric disorder such as depression or obsessive-compulsive disorder.

If you feel emotionally overwhelmed, unable to cope with your illness or with life in general, or unable to manage your usual responsibilities, treatment by a psychologist or psychiatrist may be necessary for your recovery. There are a number of psychiatric disorders, but *depression* is one of the most common, as well as one of the most treatable.

Depression can start "out of nowhere," or it can follow a stressful life event. People often talk about being "depressed" when they feel sad or discouraged. But a mental health diagnosis of depression (clinical depression) involves more than a down mood, and it's less likely to go away even after the stressful event is over. Clinical depression, unlike normal sadness or grief, includes physical and mental symptoms that make it hard to feel good or get things done. Some symptoms of depression are:

- Feeling sad *most of the time*
- Low energy and/or sleeping much more than usual
- Irritability, worry, or difficulty falling or staying asleep
- Frequent crying spells
- Loss of appetite (or overeating)
- Feelings of hopelessness or worthlessness
- Poor concentration and difficulty making decisions
- Thoughts of death or suicide

A person who has several of these symptoms lasting for more than a couple of weeks could be depressed and should be evaluated by a mental health professional. Clinical depression is a serious illness; it can interfere with recovery from medical procedures, cloud your thinking and reasoning abilities, make it more difficult to take care of your health, disrupt family relationships, and even lead to suicide. So it's very important to identify and treat it as early as possible. Fortunately, depression is usually responsive to treatment with psychotherapy, antidepressant medications, or a combination of both, and most people get better after an episode of depression. The coping techniques discussed earlier in this chapter, in combination with professional treatment, can help with recovery from depression. Regular exercise, relaxation, and social support are particularly helpful.

Professional mental health intervention is also helpful for other emotional problems that interfere with your ability to enjoy or manage your daily life, such as debilitating anxiety or panic attacks, obsessive thoughts, or dependence on alcohol or drugs. If you are experiencing these types of problems, don't just chalk it up to the stress of HHT. Get some professional help.

What's Next?

In this chapter, we've looked at coping with HHT primarily from an *individual* perspective. But HHT also affects relationships with parents, siblings, partners, and children. In the next chapter, we'll look at HHT from a *family* perspective, including communicating with your family about HHT, starting a family, teaching your children about HHT, and caring for a partner or parent who has HHT.

Chapter 5

Taking Care of Your Family

Relating to Parents and Siblings and Raising the Next Generation with HHT

Like most chronic diseases, HHT has an impact not only on the person who has it but on his or her family as well. Nonaffected family members share the feelings of frustration and loss experienced by their spouse, sibling, or child who has HHT and sometimes need to provide extra care or assume more household responsibilities when the person with HHT is ill. In many families, multiple people have HHT, compounding the impact on the family. Each person with HHT has concerns about other family members who have (or might have) it, adding to the person's worries about his or her own health. These concerns are heightened when other family members do not get tested for HHT, yet many newly diagnosed individuals find it hard to engage their families in a frank discussion of HHT and its potential consequences for the whole family.

This chapter looks at how to talk to your family of origin (parents and siblings) and other relatives to help them accept HHT as a fact of life and take action to stay healthy; how to ease the grieving process after the death of a family member from HHT-related complications; and questions to consider when you have HHT and you're thinking about having children of your own. We'll discuss becoming a parent, how you can teach your children about HHT, and what you can do to promote their health and success at school and in life. Finally, we'll talk about being the partner of someone who has HHT and how to take care of yourself while helping your partner and children live with HHT.

The plus side of having a family illness is that you are not alone. You can always look to one another for empathy and encouragement. Members of your family can work together and share their experiences and knowledge. HHT may bring you and your family closer, sharpen your appreciation for the good times you have together, and give you a chance to reevaluate what is most important to you. But first you have to get everyone to recognize that HHT is a family problem, and that's not always easy.

Telling Your Family about HHT

> We never really talked about the disease; it was just something we had. When my family sat down for the first time to really talk about HHT, I had no idea of the gravity of how my family had been affected. It really sparked something in me. We traced the line of HHT from my great-grandmother, who had nosebleeds, to my grandfather, who has GI bleeding, to my mother and uncle, and finally to me and my brother. If you don't educate others about this disease, it's just going to spiral. It's our responsibility to start the conversation.   —*Sadie*

If you're the first person in your family to be diagnosed with HHT and you're an adult, it falls to you to raise the subject. But telling your family members about their HHT "legacy," prompting them to get screened and treated, and dealing with everyone's emotional reactions can be challenging.

There are a number of different ways to communicate about HHT with your family. For example, you could give an HHT presentation to an extended family gathering or reunion. Or you could send out an e-mail or snail mail "blast" to all your family members, telling them about your diagnosis of HHT and explaining what that means for them. This may get the information out to the greatest number of people most efficiently, but a more personal approach, talking to each family member individually, can be most effective in helping them understand their risks for HHT and what they need to do about it. Talking to family members individually allows you to tailor your message to each one based on his or her age and ability to understand HHT, his or her role in the family, or your insight about what is most important in his or her life.

Before you talk to your family, give *yourself* a pep talk. Remind yourself that you are telling your family about HHT so that they can prevent disasters and stay healthy. You might even save the life of one or more of them. In other words, although you have to deliver bad news, you are doing a good deed.

You might think of yourself as an HHT ambassador. You will have more success with your family if you follow the frightening news about having HHT with a supply of resources to help them deal with it. Take brochures, fact sheets, and referral information with you, and be prepared to answer many questions. Talk first to those closest to you—your parents, siblings, and children. Later you can branch out, possibly recruiting your immediate family members to act as co-ambassadors, informing all the aunts, uncles, cousins, nieces, and nephews on the "HHT side" of your family.

As I have stressed, knowing you have HHT and making sure that your family knows about it are the keys to getting proper treatment and preventing medical disasters. So when you tell family members about HHT, it's reasonable to think they'll be grateful for this potentially life-saving news and make plans to get screened as soon as possible. But, alas, people often do not behave in a reasonable way. Some family members may feel guilt or shame about a having a genetic "defect," blame one another (and you), or blame themselves for passing HHT on to you even though they didn't know they had it. Putting these reactions aside, it's surprising how many families just don't believe that HHT can cause serious problems for them if they are not diagnosed and treated. In spite of whatever information you provide to the contrary, many family members think, "If I don't have any symptoms, I must not have HHT." And so they proceed to do absolutely nothing about it.

Denial

> As soon as I got diagnosed, I told my mom and she got screened for HHT. But my brother, who had no symptoms, refused to get tested. He had two daughters and it really frightened me to think one of his beautiful girls could get a brain abscess or a stroke—but he wouldn't budge. He's very smart, but he talked himself into thinking that if he didn't have any symptoms, he wasn't at risk. Later I told all my cousins and only one of them talked to a doctor—the others didn't think it was important and ignored the whole thing.   —*Sharon*

In Sharon's family, there was no history of sudden death or disability from HHT, nothing to scare her asymptomatic family members into getting tested. Yet even in families in which there are such tragedies or in which multiple members have nosebleeds or other symptoms, family members may not get tested.

> I have two grown daughters who refuse to get tested for HHT. They both have nosebleeds and red spots on their face and hands. And they both have kids—my grandkids!—and they won't test them either. I'm pretty sure one granddaughter has it; she's had nosebleeds since she was a baby. I don't know how to talk sense into them! I'm afraid they won't take it seriously until someone has a stroke. —*Maria*

Maria had other relatives with severe complications from HHT, and her children (and grandchildren) had nosebleeds. But despite these warning signs and Maria's pleading, her adult children would not get screened for HHT. They were in denial. We all use denial at times to protect ourselves from anxiety. It can help us cope in situations over which we have no personal control, such as being a passenger on an airplane. With HHT, there *are* some things we can do to reduce our risk of getting hurt, but denial interferes with understanding the risk, making it less likely that someone will take the actions necessary to protect himself or herself. Unfortunately, many people find their family's denial both frustrating and frightening and don't know what to do about it.

> My half-brother who's in his forties started getting a lot of nosebleeds. And my uncle and cousin get nosebleeds all the time. I've told them to get tested, but they're stubborn! They're adults, and you can't make them do it. —*Joy*

There are several things you can do to break through your family's denial and help them hear the news about HHT in a way that will inspire them to take care of themselves:

- *Set a good example.* Tell them how hard it was for you to hear about your diagnosis, what you've done about it so far, and how your actions are likely to be effective in keeping you healthy.
- *Express your love.* Tell them how much you care about them and that you're sharing the news because you want them to stay healthy too.
- *Give them information.* Give them resources such as handouts that explain the genetics of HHT as well as its major complications.
- *Emphasize prevention.* Give them some examples of medical tragedies that could have been prevented with proper treatment.

- *Give them hope.* Tell them about new treatments for HHT and promising research studies.
- *Be persistent.* If your family doesn't "get it" the first time, continue the conversation another time (and as many times after that as necessary).

Guilt, Shame, and Blame

> My Mom found out she had HHT after I got diagnosed. I was in my 30's and very anemic, and my little son had nosebleeds most days. Mom never had any symptoms, so there was no way she could have known she had HHT, but when she found out she "gave us" HHT, she was wracked with guilt. She cried and said she was sorry and that it was all her fault.   —*Sharon*

Parents tend to feel responsible for everything that happens to their children, so it's not surprising that some parents—and grandparents—feel guilty for passing HHT on to their family. Adults who find out that they have HHT any time after marriage may feel guilty about possibly burdening their spouse or partner with their illness, whether they have symptoms or anticipate future problems. And anyone diagnosed with HHT who has to tell his or her family about it may feel guilty just being the bearer of bad news. Even though you know your family members should be screened, you may feel guilty when screening reveals lung or brain AVMs.

Guilt in these situations is emotional, not rational. So if you or a family member is struggling with guilt, remind yourself—or them—to challenge this feeling. Focusing on rational thoughts about HHT and its impact on the family can help ease painful guilt feelings. Here are a few examples:

- HHT is nobody's fault. It's a random genetic mutation.
- I didn't choose to give my children HHT. I had no control over which genes I passed on.
- It's good (not bad) that my family member found out about a lung AVM, because now she can get treated and avoid a stroke.
- I can help my child learn how to manage HHT and live a good life.
- My partner and I made a commitment to take care of each other in sickness and in health. That includes HHT.

In some families, illness is experienced as a source of shame. Although many people in our society speak openly about cancer and other serious medical conditions, shame and secrecy about illness still exist. Shame is influenced by cultural and family beliefs, personality traits, and individual life experiences.

> My grandfather had constant nosebleeds and died of a "heart attack" in his 40's. Even if his family knew about HHT, Italian immigrants in the early 1900s would never admit to such a "defect." My cousin refused to admit she had this disease because she thought it would "taint" her children. Her brother has heavy nosebleeds, but stoically does not complain.   —Rhoda

In Rhoda's family, shame led to hiding HHT, discouraging family members from getting diagnosed, and rejecting much-needed medical care. Being "stoic" about symptoms and suffering in silence was seen as preferable to admitting a "defect" but resulted in familywide ignorance about HHT and several disastrous medical consequences.

If you experience shame or humiliation related to your genetic "defect" or your symptoms of HHT, try to get support from people outside your immediate family, who can give you a different perspective. Think about the positive consequences of openness about your HHT—getting support from others, getting proper treatment, helping your family, and the chance to feel proud of yourself for "coming out of the closet." You may want to seek confidential help from a mental health professional or genetic counselor to conquer feelings of shame and begin taking better care of yourself.

The flip side of feeling guilt and shame is blaming (or shaming) someone else. Some family members want to "shoot the messenger"; they blame you for bringing them news about HHT and get angry. Or they shame you for being a "complainer" or "weakling." Their expressions of anger or contempt can prompt you to get defensive or angry yourself, and before long you've got a real family tussle. Try to avoid defensive reactions whenever possible by staying rational and "on script" with your family, reminding yourself that it's not your fault (or anyone's) and reminding your family that you told them about HHT because you love them and want them to be healthy and safe.

Coping with Grief

There are multiple losses associated with HHT, but the death of loved ones from HHT-related illness is the most emotionally painful. Grieving after a death is a normal process, one that typically becomes more manageable over time. Feelings of profound loss, distress, and disorientation recede gradually, and special memories of the loved one or valuable lessons learned from him or her become more prominent. Talking to family members about shared losses, finding a way to honor your loved one who has died, expressing your feelings in a journal or poem, and having an annual ritual to remember your loved one are some ways to cope with grief. Some people find that donating to HHT research, volunteering, or becoming an advocate for others with HHT is a meaningful way to honor the memory of a loved one who died from HHT.

Support from outside the family can be helpful too. Many hospitals, hospice centers, and religious congregations offer grief support groups, usually led by trained volunteers. Groups use structured discussions, writing or artwork, and sharing feelings with others in the group to guide people through normal grieving.

People in mourning are usually able to get back into the normal routines of life after several months. They may remain sad or cry when thinking or talking about the death of their loved one, but they are able to enjoy other relationships and activities (like playing with a grandchild, having dinner with a friend, working, and so forth). But sometimes people get "stuck" in grieving and become clinically depressed. If, after the loss of a loved one, you are deeply sad or hopeless about life in general, are unable to manage day-to-day activities, or find yourself isolated from your usual social contacts, consider seeking help from a mental health professional.

Partnering and Parenting with HHT

Telling Your Romantic Partner about HHT

I was not diagnosed with HHT until after I was married. At which point, I asked my wife if she'd like a divorce, allowing her to escape this arduous journey that I was embarking upon. Thankfully, she declined and has been a gift from God ever since, providing both love and emotional balance.   —*Lenny*

Until fairly recently, many people married and had children before they knew they had HHT. HHT was an "uninvited guest" in their life and in their marriage. Spouses like Lenny's were surprised by the diagnosis of HHT in their loved ones and had to make the best of it. What if Lenny's wife had known about his HHT *before* marriage? Would she have chosen not to marry him? As more people with HHT are being diagnosed at a younger age, they wonder how a potential spouse or partner will feel about their HHT and when and how they should tell dating partners that they have HHT.

HHT is not something you need to discuss on the first date if you don't want to, although if you have a nosebleed, you might want to be up-front about what's going on. And if you are someone who's comfortable talking matter-of-factly about medical problems, there's no reason *not* to talk about it on the first date. In fact, some people prefer to "put their cards on the table" right away, not wanting to get involved with anyone who would see HHT as a reason not to date further.

If you have serious symptoms of HHT, it may be hard to keep it from your boyfriend or girlfriend for very long. Telling your partner about your HHT may be a way to deepen your friendship and intimacy.

I'm dating someone now and he supports me, he knows all about it. It wasn't hard to talk to him. I told him to look up HHT on the Internet and he did and he said he was sorry I had it. He knows my health issues and he plans to hang out with me after my procedure.

—*Nicole*

It's possible that some dates or potential partners will not want to continue a romantic relationship once they know about your HHT. But others will see your HHT as "part of the package," something they willingly accept because they want to be with *you.*

If you haven't told your partner about HHT, it's probably a good idea to share this part of your life as you move into a "serious" relationship. Because you have a genetic illness that could affect your health in dramatic and unpredictable ways and be passed along to your children, the person who will be your life partner and coparent should know about this condition. Telling your partner specifics about how HHT affects your current health and what symptoms you anticipate in future years can help him or her understand what you are dealing with—and decide whether to go "all in" with you. Make sure your partner gets educated about HHT by reading this book, visiting the Cure HHT website, and/or attending a patient-and-family conference.

In addition to sharing the facts of HHT, you and your partner will benefit from honest discussions of your beliefs and expectations about how illness, disability, and caregiving might affect your relationship. If you are uncertain whether HHT might prevent you from fully committing to your relationship, you may want to seek premarital couples counseling to clarify your feelings and make the best decision.

Becoming a Parent: Whether to Pass on HHT

> I am currently in a serious relationship and have been with my partner for six years, so naturally we have talked about having children. Passing on the HHT gene is a significant concern for both of us. My symptoms are currently an inconvenience—a five-minute nosebleed once a week—and with the variability of the disease, it's hard to predict the future of offspring with HHT. Family planning is not in our immediate future, but I do have the number for a geneticist at the HHT Center, for when that time arrives.   —*Sadie*

Today's young adults who know they have HHT have more choices available to them than previous generations did. In the past, most people didn't get diagnosed until well after their children were born; and for those who did, the technology enabling a choice of whether to pass on the HHT gene was not developed. If you plan to have children, you and your partner (or fiancée) might want to discuss your options with a genetic counselor and your personal physician. While many prospective parents continue to take their chances with regard to possibly passing HHT on to their children, reproductive technologies now exist to *prevent* passing it on. These technologies, however, are not an option for *all* prospective parents, because they pose some health risks for the mother and the unborn child. They are also very expensive, raising ethical concerns about class discrimination (wealthy prospective parents can afford not to have children with genetic disorders, but low-income prospective parents often don't have this option) and moral concerns about abortion and the destruction of embryos (see below). Such concerns may rule out the use of these technologies for some people. Prospective parents can choose to adopt children if they feel very strongly about not passing on HHT but don't want to, or can't afford to, use reproduction technologies.

Because of family experiences of suffering or disability from HHT, some prospective parents feel strongly that it would be unfair to bring a child with HHT into the world. For them, if they can afford it, the benefits of having a biological child who does not have HHT may be worth the risks and expenses associated with the use of reproductive technology.

> After years of putting off pregnancy, I started noticing programs and news articles about the advances made in IVF [in vitro fertilization]. I realized there was a chance I could have children without them inheriting my HHT gene. I inquired further with my genetics doctor and she confirmed this can be done. I was ecstatic.   —*Jane*

So what is possible? First, genetic testing for HHT can be done on the fetus, while a woman is pregnant; this is called *prenatal genetic testing*. This is done using one of two procedures: either *chorionic villus sampling (CVS)*, between the tenth and thirteenth weeks of pregnancy, or *amniocentesis*, between the fifteenth and twentieth weeks. CVS uses a sample of tissue from the placenta, while amniocentesis uses a sample of the amniotic fluid (both the placenta and amniotic fluid contain cells containing the genes of the fetus). With amniocentesis, the tissue sample is extracted by inserting a long, thin needle into the woman's abdomen. With CVS, the same method may be used, or the sample may be extracted through the woman's cervix. To prevent bearing a child that tests positive for HHT, termination of the pregnancy (that is, an abortion) would be necessary if the fetus were found to have a mutation associated with HHT, and the parents would need to repeat the test with each pregnancy until they conceived a child without HHT. These procedures are uncomfortable for the mother, and they slightly increase her risk for a miscarriage. Having multiple abortions also carries medical and psychological risks.

Another effective procedure that can ensure that a child will not have HHT is *preimplantation genetic diagnosis (PGD)* combined with *in vitro fertilization (IVF)*. This is a difficult procedure, but it does not require terminating a pregnancy. In IVF, a procedure used by many infertile couples, eggs are removed from the woman's ovaries and combined with the man's sperm in a laboratory. Typically, many embryos are created and several are implanted in the woman's uterus, while the rest are saved for possible future use. Using PGD, the embryos are tested for HHT *before* any are implanted. Only the embryos that do not carry the genetic mutation for HHT are implanted, while embryos that test positive for HHT are destroyed.

IVF is very expensive, although some insurance companies may cover part of the cost (the amount varies widely among insurance companies). IVF also involves moderate physical discomfort and health risks for the woman and can be challenging emotionally for both parents. Sometimes the process fails to produce a pregnancy and has to be repeated. Sometimes the procedure results in multiple births, since several embryos are placed in the uterus to increase the chances of a pregnancy. However, for couples who do not want their children to inherit HHT, this is an option to consider.

> All in all, this process can be quite draining, emotional and expensive, but the relief of knowing the HHT gene stops with me is a feeling I cannot describe. I hope other women with HHT or other life-threatening genetic disorders will also consider IVF as an option.
>
> —*Jane*

Prenatal and preimplantation genetic testing raise questions about whether it is reasonable, ethical, or moral to terminate a pregnancy or destroy embryos in order to prevent having a child with HHT. The weight of risks versus benefits makes these techniques somewhat controversial for *any* genetic disease, but many people believe their use is justified when the gene in question always results in a life of extreme suffering or severe disability. Because the severity of HHT is highly variable and most people who know they have HHT can live satisfying lives, these techniques are not widely used in the HHT community. This may change in the future as the technologies are refined and perhaps made less expensive, safer, or easier for parents.

Use of reproductive technologies is a highly personal decision, best made with the guidance of an obstetrician, a primary care physician, and a genetic counselor to help you weigh the anticipated impacts of HHT on your child against the risks, expenses, and discomforts associated with prenatal genetic testing or IVF and PGD. Your genetic counselor can help ensure that the choice you make is the right one for you.

Parenting a Child with HHT

Many people diagnosed with HHT before becoming parents are willing to accept the 50 percent chance of passing it on to their children. Parents who know they have HHT and have been properly screened, treated, and educated about HHT know they can greatly reduce their children's risk of serious complications and increase the likelihood that their children with HHT will have fulfilling lives.

As discussed in earlier chapters, the most important thing parents with HHT can do to ensure the health of their children is to get them screened as soon as possible so as to reduce the risk of complications from lung and brain AVMs. Beyond that, parents can play an essential part in educating their children about HHT, advocating for their needs, and supporting them so that they develop a positive attitude toward life.

> I want what all parents want—for our kids to have healthy, long lives filled with spontaneity and life. —*Donnie*

If you know you have HHT before you become a parent and decide to let nature take its course, you have time to prepare for the possibility of having a child with HHT. You can read up on the latest recommendations for screening and treatments in children and get genetic counseling if you have questions. You might consider having the genetic test for HHT so that your baby can have genetic testing early in life and potentially avoid expensive and stressful clinical screenings. Lung AVMs and most brain AVMs are too small to be detected while a baby is still in utero, but an ultrasound during the pregnancy may be able to detect a very large brain AVM in the fetus. This information could be useful in planning for a safe delivery and specialized prenatal medical care. Genetic testing can also be done soon after birth, using blood from the umbilical cord. If you would like to have this option, make sure to tell your obstetrician or midwife before the baby is delivered.

Coping with the Diagnosis of HHT in Your Child

Even when you know there's a 50 percent chance that *each* of your children will have HHT, you may be surprised if *all* of your children inherit HHT. Similarly, you may know all about your own symptoms of HHT but be caught off guard if your child's manifestations of HHT are more severe than your own. Maybe you "knew" your child could have a brain AVM, but some part of your mind didn't really believe it was possible since no one else in your family had ever had one. If your child does have a brain AVM or some other serious complication, not only is it frightening but it may create or intensify feelings of guilt about passing HHT on to your child. You may experience self-blame, anxiety, or a sense of personal failure. These feelings may be unavoidable and seem very real and distressing, but you can conquer them with emotional support and by focusing on solving the problem at hand, namely, taking care of your child.

> I will never forget that feeling of shock and panic after hearing that all three of my children tested positive for HHT. I'd thought that one probably had it because of her nightly nosebleeds, and possibly the other, who is currently nosebleed free but has six telltale telangiectasias on her hands. Though my third child had also had a few nosebleeds, I held out hope that at least one of my children had escaped this heartbreaking diagnosis. Within 24 hours of finding out that my daughters had HHT and one night of little sleep, I decided that they had to undergo the screening process.   —*Lorna*

Lorna quickly moved through the stages many parents experience, albeit over a longer period of time: hoping against hope that their child won't get HHT (or have complications from it); feeling shocked and heartbroken when their children develop symptoms and are diagnosed with HHT; and ultimately resolving to take care of their children in the best way they possibly can.

If you are a parent who has HHT, you may already have a good support system in place—friends or family who give you an emotional boost at stressful times. Support from other family members, friends, or the HHT community (through online support, grass-roots HHT groups, or HHT patient and family conferences) is especially important when your child is diagnosed with HHT, has a medical complication, or needs to be in the hospital. Having someone who can give you a break, cheer you up, or let you vent will help you cope with your emotions and focus on taking care of your child.

Teaching Your Child about HHT

> Have faith, have patience. And get all the information you can
> about HHT.   —Robin

The current medical recommendation to parents who have HHT is to screen their children for HHT early in life, if possible with genetic testing first and then with a variety of clinical tests, depending on whether the child is symptomatic. It's equally important to teach your child about HHT, and it's never too early to start. (Sometimes a young child is the first to be diagnosed in a family, because of a serious complication or because of frequent nosebleeds. When this happens, the parents will need to be screened for HHT and educate themselves. You may be just one chapter ahead of your child, but you can begin passing on information about HHT.)

It's helpful to focus on teaching your child to manage the symptoms— whether nosebleeds, fatigue, or disability from a stroke—that are affecting his or her life at the time. Ask your child's HHT doctor about anything you don't understand regarding your child's symptoms or about HHT in general. Then try to answer your child's questions honestly but simply. Use words your child can understand. For example, if a 4-year-old needs treatment for a brain AVM, you might want to tell him that he has a "boo-boo" in his head and reassure him that the doctor can fix it while he's sleeping; for an older child, you might add a simple explanation of an AVM (abnormal blood vessels that can bleed unexpectedly) and more details about preparing for the procedure and about what happens during recovery; for a teenager, you could go a step further by explaining the risks and benefits of treatment and providing more technical details on how the procedure is done.

Try not to overwhelm your child with information about unlikely events, such as liver or GI involvement, which may not happen until the child is much older, if ever. You can tell your child more about the less common manifestations of HHT as he or she matures or if you or others in the family begin to experience them. If you gradually give your child more education and allow the child more input in decisions about his or her care, your child will begin to take more responsibility and become more competent at managing his or her own health as he or she enters the teen years and young adulthood. One of the best ways to teach your middle-school and older children how to manage HHT is by being a good role model and making sure your kids know what you're doing to take care of your own HHT.

Advocating for Your Child

Anything for my daughter, I will do it.   —*Robin*

There are many situations in which you may need to advocate for your child with teachers, doctors, and other adults who interact with him or her, including parents of the child's friends. Let them know about your child's HHT-related needs and what they can do to help. Insist that your doctors become informed about HHT if they are unfamiliar with it. To help your child succeed at school and manage his or her HHT, you can request *accommodations*, such as extra time to complete classwork or homework, rest breaks during gym class (or *no* gym class), permission to leave class to attend to nosebleeds, or other adjustments in routines depending on whether your child's HHT affects his or her energy, thinking, breathing, or mobility.

The Americans with Disabilities Act (ADA), the same law that provides for accommodations in the workplace, protects children from educational discrimination and ensures that all children have equal access to *public* schooling regardless of disability. (This part of the ADA law is called Section 504.) Public schools must provide reasonable accommodations so that your child with HHT can get the same quality education as any other child. (Though *private* schools are exempt from the ADA, many will make a good-faith effort to meet your child's needs.)

Parents can begin the process of getting accommodations for their child by requesting a meeting with the school administrator to create an Individualized Education Program (IEP) or 504 Plan for their child. Parents should put their request in writing as well; a letter can be mailed to the administrator, or you can take it with you to the meeting. If possible, take a letter from your child's doctor explaining how HHT affects your child and suggesting specific accommodations. The school staff may ask for additional medical information or evaluations in order to help them make the best plan. The school should involve the parents in all steps of the planning process.

Involving your child in advocacy and awareness events can bolster the child's confidence and improve his or her ability to communicate clearly with other children and adults about HHT and their needs. The earlier they practice these skills, the more they'll be able to speak up for themselves when they're adults.

> I used to get embarrassed by nosebleeds at friends' houses. Now I always tell my new friends about HHT. I like to talk to people, to get it off my head, it helps to share it. I talk to teachers, my mom, friends—my whole school knows about me! Everyone asks how I am today, and I always tell them. And I was in a video they made at the children's hospital where I went for my lung AVMs.   —*Nicole*

Fostering a Positive Attitude

You can help your child learn to cope with the impact of HHT on his social life, such as playdates with friends, sports activities, sleepovers, and dating. Kids can benefit from the same coping strategies adults use, such as adapting social activities to fit their abilities. If they don't have the energy for sports or physical play, they can play board games, draw, or watch movies with their friends. And they can learn to set their own priorities (with some guidance from parents), deciding which activities are most important and setting aside less important ones.

You can help your child do some reframing too. Praise him when he's done well in managing his symptoms or in handling the stress of a hospital test or procedure. Telling your child that he or she is brave, calm, a strong person, or good at solving problems will help the child feel self-confident and proud. Try to emphasize your child's strengths and capabilities rather than focusing on his or her nosebleeds or energy limitations.

> My daughter's had six AVMs coiled in one lung, and she has three more in the other lung and one in her brain that will need treatment

soon. But she keeps up with her friends and we do a lot of fun things together. She did a fundraiser and we'll be at the next HHT walk. She is a tower of strength!   —*Robin*

Teach your child not to focus excessively on his nosebleeds or other symptoms of HHT. Encourage the child to play, socialize, and have as normal a life as possible. When talking with your child's teachers, parents of the child's friends, or other adults, stress that aside from having HHT, your child is just like other children. When you consistently present your child in a positive light, your child develops greater self-esteem and learns that HHT is just one part of his or her life. Most children with HHT are able to cope quite well. Regular play and exercise, relaxation, and friendships will help them manage stress and have a positive outlook. But children may have periods of emotional distress when they are ill or need a procedure or are concerned about illness in a parent or other family member. Professional counseling by a school psychologist or guidance counselor can help your child cope with sadness, anxiety, or feeling left out or "different" because of HHT. If your child seems depressed, hopeless, or excessively anxious, aggressive, or isolated from other children, seek help from a child psychologist or psychiatrist. Children and teenagers can become depressed and even suicidal. If your child expresses any thoughts about suicide, take it seriously and get help right away.

Caregivers in HHT Families

My fiancé had surgery for a brain abscess, but then he bled excessively, causing a stroke—and after almost a year in the hospital, nursing homes, and rehabilitation, he is now 26 years old, disabled, in a wheelchair, and being cared for by me at home. I am his girlfriend, caregiver, advocate, therapist, housewife, you name it!   —*Karen*

Caregivers for adults with disabilities or chronic illness are most often the person's spouse/partner or adult child. Some adults with HHT need help from a family caregiver because they have limited energy or mobility caused by anemia, heart failure, stroke, or other complications. Family caregivers may provide emotional support and act as advocates or surrogate decision makers when their partner or parent with HHT is ill or disabled. They may provide hands-on care such as help with bathing or dressing or help a person do their home physical therapy exercises. They may act as "accessory brains," helping their spouse or parent to remember things, reason out problems, or keep medical information organized.

Caregiving can be physically exhausting and emotionally stressful. Karen's experience of wearing multiple hats and doing virtually everything for her fiancé is one shared by many caregivers, especially spouses or partners. Caregivers can easily become overwhelmed, depressed, or socially isolated. But proper support and education can make caregiving much easier. Here are some tips to help "nonaffected" caregivers stay on track:

- *Educate yourself.* Learn enough about your loved one's needs so you can be an advocate and a hands-on caregiver.
- *Don't overdo it.* Let your loved one do as much for herself or himself as possible. Overprotecting can make the ill person feel useless or guilty about needing help.
- *Take care of yourself too.* Take rest breaks, get enough sleep, eat well, exercise, and attend to your own health needs.
- *Get emotional support.* Join a caregiver support group (many hospitals and community centers offer these groups) and keep in touch with close friends and family.
- *Take care of your relationship.* Don't let illness and caregiving overshadow your expressions of affection, friendship, or intimacy.
- *Have a backup plan.* Line up someone who can care for your loved one if you are unavailable.
- *Attend to legal matters.* Make sure you have power of attorney, a health care proxy, a will, a living will, or any other documents you need so you can easily act on your loved one's behalf in an emergency or if he or she is incapacitated. An attorney can help you make sure your papers are in order.
- *Get help with depression.* If you feel depressed, get help from a mental health professional.

What's Next?

The prior chapter dealt with *individual* coping skills to reduce HHT's impact on emotions and quality of life. This chapter broadened the lens to include management of HHT in *family* life—communication, parenting, and caregiving. In the next chapter, we'll look beyond individual people and their families to see what steps can be taken in the broader social world to make life better for *everyone* affected by HHT. We'll look at how you can help conquer obstacles by becoming an advocate for better access to medical care, greater awareness of HHT, and legislative support and fundraising for HHT research and treatment.

Chapter 6

Beyond the Family
Conquering Obstacles with Advocacy

> Patients *must* be their own advocates. They should arm all of their
> physicians with knowledge about HHT. —*Sadie*

Being an advocate means standing up for your own rights and taking
action to get your needs met or helping others to do the same. Because HHT
is an uncommon disorder, is hard to diagnose, and has received limited
federal funding, people with HHT can benefit from acting as advocates for
themselves and others with the disorder. Some goals of advocacy include
increasing awareness about HHT among doctors, the public, and lawmakers; ensuring adequate funding for HHT research to develop the best possible treatments; and increasing access to high-quality medical care.

Advocacy has practical and psychological benefits. The more effectively
you advocate for yourself or your family, the more successful you'll be in
getting what you need. Using coping strategies such as reframing, relax-
ing, and talking to friends can help you manage your emotional responses
to HHT and start to feel better. But when you become an advocate, even
by doing something as simple as giving your child's school nurse an HHT
fact sheet, you are taking another significant step on your own behalf and
on behalf of others with HHT. Advocacy focuses on problems; it helps you
cope by taking action to solve a problem, potentially reducing not only your
stress but also the source of your stress (in this example, once the school
nurse knows about HHT, you won't have to worry about what will happen
when your child gets a nosebleed at school).

Advocacy can give your life more purpose and enhance your sense of
effectiveness in the world. Advocacy also brings you into contact with more
people in your community, creating valuable networks of social support.
Finally, being an advocate is a recognized and respected social role, a way
of participating in the world that is valued by others. And with the help of

computers and the Internet, you can be an advocate even if you are physically limited by HHT-related health problems.

Medical Advocacy

Even when you and your family are in the know about HHT and ready to do what it takes to stay healthy, there may be external obstacles to getting the best treatment possible. Interactions with medical, insurance, and benefit systems can be challenging. Acting as your own advocate will help you avoid falling through the cracks.

Insurance Coverage

> Once diagnosed with HHT, your family is in for a really tough time. My two brothers and my four children all had to get tested for HHT. These tests are not cheap, and it's like pulling teeth to get your insurance company to pay for them when your family members haven't been diagnosed with anything yet!   —*Tom*

Many people confront obstacles to getting insurance coverage for HHT screening tests or for genetic testing. Insurance policies and coverage rules are often hard to understand, and different representatives of your insurance company may give you conflicting information about what is and is not covered. Read your insurance manual carefully. If your insurance is through your employer, you may be able to get help understanding your coverage from someone in your employee benefits department.

Some insurance companies assign *case managers* to help people with chronic illnesses stay well. Although they are employed by the insurance company, case managers usually advocate for the patient, creating a win-win situation: the insurance company provides coverage for tests and treatment that can prevent very expensive medical disasters such as a stroke, which would cost the company much more than the preventive tests and treatments, so the company saves money and you stay healthy. If you are not offered the services of a case manager, you can ask your insurance company whether it provides this service.

Most insurance providers, including Medicare, will eventually agree to cover HHT-related care, including genetic testing, but it can be difficult and confusing to deal directly with your insurance company. Another way to get around insurance obstacles is to find a doctor or an HHT Center of Excellence whose staff can advocate for insurance coverage on your behalf. Insurance companies may require a referral from your primary care doctor, letters from your HHT doctors, and diagnostic and procedure codes that only a medical office can supply. Before you waste time and energy fighting your insurance company, ask your providers if they can handle this for you. Most HHT Centers of Excellence, genetic counselors, and genetic testing labs will communicate with your insurance company to make sure it covers genetic testing for HHT. There is good evidence that genetic testing costs less than doing clinical HHT screening on every at-risk family member, evidence that insurance companies may take into consideration.

Finally, if your insurance company seems to be stonewalling your efforts to get care, you can contact the insurance commissioner in your state for assistance. You can find the name and contact information for your state's insurance commissioner at the website for the National Association of Insurance Commissioners, www.naic.org/documents/members _membershiplist.pdf (see the "Resources" section for full contact information). The office of the commissioner can help you understand your coverage and negotiate with your insurance company. If your insurance company is restricting your coverage inappropriately, the commissioner's office will help you file a formal complaint and then investigate and take action on your behalf.

In the past, people worried that an official diagnosis of HHT would result in discrimination by insurance companies, especially that they would lose coverage because of a preexisting condition. Since the passage of the Affordable Care Act (ACA), which eliminated the use of preexisting conditions as a reason to deny insurance coverage, this has not been a concern in the United States. A law called the Genetic Information Nondiscrimination Act (GINA) has been in effect even longer than the ACA and states that insurance companies can't use your genetic information (such as a family history of HHT) to deny insurance coverage. However, both these laws may be altered significantly in the coming years; it is important to be aware of how changes in these laws or new health care legislation might affect your insurance coverage and to consider advocating with Congress in favor of protecting coverage for people with genetic diseases and chronic health conditions.

Specialty Medical Care for HHT

Sometimes it's difficult for people to obtain a referral to an HHT Center of Excellence or a doctor who specializes in HHT care. With some health insurance plans (and in some countries outside the United States), your primary care doctor acts as a gatekeeper; that is, you are required to get a referral from him or her in order for your insurance to pay for your care at a specialty center or hospital. If you must advocate for a referral, provide your doctor with written information about HHT (the Cure HHT handout for physicians is a good overview) and tell him or her about the Cure HHT website. Request that your doctor consult with a staff person at Cure HHT and with the medical director or clinic coordinator at the HHT Center of Excellence where you would like to be treated. If possible, take a family member or friend with you to support your request.

> It can be incredibly difficult to get your family doctor to send you for HHT screening. So many doctors are hesitant to make the referral—maybe they think it's not necessary or they think it's too expensive. I'm glad I convinced my doctor to give me the referral for screening at an HHT Center. I had to bring him a ton of information from the Internet and then actually *demand* that he send me to the Center. I told him I wouldn't leave his office until he gave me the referral! When your life is at stake, you have to be a little pushy.   —*Linda*

At the HHT Center of Excellence, Linda's screening revealed a small brain AVM. Linda knew that HHT was in her family. By advocating for herself—and for her young son—she was able to get an accurate diagnosis and treatment for all of them.

While there are an increasing number of HHT Centers of Excellence around the country, there are still areas in the United States and elsewhere where distance from the nearest center makes travel to and from them burdensome. You may be able to find a local doctor with some HHT experience through the physician directory on the Cure HHT website. But if you live in a rural area, you may not find anyone in your community who knows about HHT. In that case, you'll have to advocate for yourself with your local doctor or hospital to make sure they understand HHT and how to treat you effectively.

It's a good idea to let your primary care doctor know as soon as you suspect or find out that you have HHT. Provide your doctor with as much educational material as you can get your hands on and ask him or her to consult with an expert for advice in managing your care. If your doctor is willing to do some homework on the Internet and make a phone call or two, he or she may be able to order screening tests at your local hospital and manage some of your HHT symptoms.

When possible, it's best to go to an HHT Center of Excellence for complex problems such as liver involvement and brain AVM treatment, as discussed earlier. But local doctors who become familiar with your symptoms, medical needs, and current treatment options for HHT are in a better position to provide emergency care for unexpected complications, as happened in Carla's case.

> Due to severe nosebleeds requiring numerous blood transfusions, I planned to have a Young's procedure done at an HHT Center of Excellence far from my home. But the surgery had to be postponed by the Center and before it could be rescheduled, I had yet another disastrous nosebleed and became too ill to travel. Although they had limited experience with Young's procedure, my ENTs realized this was the only way to prevent another life-threatening nosebleed, so they decided to do the Young's procedure at the local hospital. Because they had become educated about HHT, they were able to save my life.   —*Carla*

While some doctors have an idea of the range of symptoms caused by HHT, their knowledge of the currently recommended screenings and treatments may be out of date, either incomplete or incorrect. So be sure that you provide your doctors with the most up-to-date information you can find. If you require a procedure such as laser treatment for nosebleeds, make sure your local doctor is using the most current techniques. You may need to contact a specialist at an HHT Center of Excellence or consult with Cure HHT to find out about the most current recommendations and then discuss them with your doctor. If your local doctor is uninterested in the information you provide or unwilling to discuss treatment options, you should think about getting a second opinion. Advocating for the best medical care includes finding doctors that accept you as their partner in your care. Experienced doctors know that listening to the patient is crucial to good medical practice. If your doctor tunes you out, it's time to find one who will listen.

Sometimes you have to go to an emergency room for a severe nosebleed or a non-HHT-related emergency. Very likely the ER doctor will know almost nothing about HHT. If so, it's important to advocate for yourself by telling ER doctors about HHT and insisting that they look at the Cure HHT website or call your doctor before doing any invasive treatments or tests. As discussed in chapter 3, you should avoid certain tests, such as liver biopsies, and certain pain medications, such as nonsteroidal anti-inflammatory (NSAID) drugs (such as Advil or Motrin), that could make your HHT worse. A legitimate concern is what happens if you are taken to an ER and are unconscious or can't speak for yourself. Wearing a *medical alert bracelet* bearing the information that you have HHT and giving the website and phone number for Cure HHT or your HHT doctor can help make sure that you get the appropriate care. Other options include carrying a wallet card with your medical information or wearing a bracelet that contains a computer data storage device containing your medical records.

Legislative Advocacy

> Legislative advocacy is the key to raising awareness about HHT and creating financial resources for the disease. It's tough work to get funding for much of anything in today's Congress, particularly disease-specific funding.
> —*Sadie*

Legislative advocacy involves communicating with your senators and congressional representatives about the needs of the HHT community, including your own needs. In recent years, legislative advocacy in the HHT community has focused on securing the passage of the Hereditary Hemorrhagic Telangiectasia Diagnosis and Treatment Act. If passed, the act would require federal funding for a coordinated effort led by the National Institutes of Health (NIH) and the Centers for Disease Control and Prevention

(CDC) to increase early diagnosis and treatment for HHT, create an HHT resource center at the CDC, and conduct public awareness programs.

> Advocacy is as much about the journey as the outcome. While advocating for a specific bill, you talk to congressional staffers and elected officials, maybe even start a petition. With each individual you speak to or each citizen who signs your petition, you create awareness. That is one more person who knows the symptoms of HHT, one more person who knows the devastating effects of the disease, one more person who knows the negative financial implications of a late diagnosis, and one more person who can make a difference.   —*Sadie*

More broadly, legislative advocacy helps to increase awareness of HHT among lawmakers and to solicit their support of HHT Centers of Excellence and hospitals that treat HHT. It is a way to give feedback to your representatives on issues such as problems with insurance coverage for HHT or difficulties accessing care. By writing letters to your representatives in Congress and visiting with them in person, you can tell them how HHT has affected your family's life. Personal stories and face-to-face meetings are an effective way to increase their awareness of HHT. Each year, Cure HHT sponsors a Capitol Hill Day. Prior to that day, Cure HHT legislative consultants and volunteers prepare people with HHT for meeting with their representatives, and then they accompany them to the meetings if needed. Participating in Capitol Hill Day is a great way to become your own legislative advocate.

Awareness and Fundraising

Awareness includes any activity you engage in to educate or inform other people about HHT. Examples include writing to your local newspaper about HHT, giving a short presentation to the nurse at your child's school, sharing your HHT story on social media or on the Cure HHT website, talking to friends and family about HHT, and so forth. Awareness events can also be used as opportunities for fundraising. These events can include, for example, walks, bike rides or other athletic events, bake sales, dances, or potluck dinners. Some people simply write a letter or e-mail telling friends about HHT and asking them to donate; there are also websites available specifically for this purpose, such as www.everydayhero.com and www .gofundme.com. Cure HHT can help you get started by supporting your ideas, publicizing your event, and linking you to a fundraising website.

What's Next?

One of the obstacles faced by people with HHT is the lack of effective treatment for some symptoms of HHT. Medical research is the key to finding these treatments, but until recently research on HHT was limited by a lack of funding. Currently, several promising HHT researchers have obtained government research grants, and pharmaceutical companies are beginning to sponsor research on drugs to treat HHT. Research will shape the future of HHT care, and there is hope that research will lead to a cure.

The final chapter describes recent and anticipated advances in HHT research in both basic science (the genetic and biochemical mechanisms of HHT) and clinical or applied science (new treatments, procedures, and technologies). It looks at how research is funded and how you can help advance progress in HHT research as a research supporter, fundraiser, or participant.

As the stories in this book make clear, people with HHT can improve their lives in many different ways—managing their physical health, coping with emotional responses to HHT, dealing with family dimensions of HHT, and becoming advocates for themselves and others. In the next chapter, you'll learn how research, and your involvement as a participant or supporter, will make life with HHT even better for future generations.

Part III

Into the Future

Chapter 7

Frontiers in HHT Research

Expanding Knowledge and Developing New Treatments

> I really want to find an answer for families in which we don't
> know why they have HHT. Research is like a roller coaster—One
> day you think you've found a new [gene] variant that causes
> HHT and the next you find that same variant in a control sample.
> We will get there though. I'm determined!
> —*Whitney Wooderchak-Donahue, PhD, HHT genetics research scientist*[1]

This is an exciting time for research on HHT. Studies that seek to
better understand the genetics of HHT and the mechanisms of AVM
formation (basic science research) and those aimed at developing new
medications, procedures, and other therapies for HHT (clinical research)
are bringing us closer than ever to a cure. We can expect that in our life-
times significant advances in HHT treatment will dramatically reduce
symptoms and improve quality of life for many people with HHT.

This chapter provides an overview of the major developments in HHT
research to date, discusses ongoing research projects, and describes new
or planned cutting-edge studies. It explains how HHT research is funded
and how you can contribute to advances in HHT research.

Basic Science Research

Basic science research looks at the *mechanisms* of HHT. It asks, for example, how AVMs form and what makes them grow; why only some vessels
are abnormal in HHT, while most are normal; why people with the same
HHT gene have different symptoms; and what genes cause HHT in families that do not have a mutation in one of the HHT genes already identified. Basic science studies do not use human beings as subjects. They
are conducted in laboratories working either with human cell or tissue

samples or with animals. The term *animal model* refers to the use of animals to study disease states, mechanisms of illness, and the effects of various drugs or procedures to treat the disease. Animal models are essential to understanding diseases and treatments and set the stage for *clinical research*, which tests the effectiveness of drugs and procedures in treating humans.

Of Mice and Men: The HHT Knock-Out Mouse

Mice are widely used for creating animal models in medical research, and HHT is no exception. You may have heard some time ago about the first "HHT knock-out mouse." This was a laboratory mouse in which researchers deactivated, or "knocked out," one of the genes involved in blood vessel formation, resulting in a mouse with HHT-like symptoms. When you read about a "mouse model of HHT," that's what it refers to: a mouse that has been genetically altered to give it HHT. Because humans and mice have many of the same genes, studying gene changes in mice can help scientists understand how these genes cause or contribute to disease in humans.

Early knock-out studies showed that mice missing one *ALK1* or one *ENG* gene (recall that a normal animal has two of each gene) reached adulthood but had some vascular abnormalities, whereas mice missing both *ALK1* genes or both *ENG* genes died in utero because of severe defects in blood vessel and heart development. Scientists are now refining these mouse models to study the effects of deactivating either *ENG* or *ALK1* genes at different times in mouse development and in different cell types in order to create HHT-like symptoms in mice that more closely resemble those in humans. These refined models also allow them to study the effects of other genes and environmental factors that influence blood vessel and AVM development. By creating mice that develop AVMs more similar to those in humans with HHT, including lung and brain AVMs, researchers can get more precise information about the causes of AVMs and generate new ideas about how to prevent or treat AVMs in humans.

Knock-out mice are routinely used for testing the effectiveness and safety of drug therapies for HHT before they are tried in humans. For example, the use of thalidomide in a mouse model led to a trial of the drug in HHT patients with severe nosebleeds, and discovery of the critical role of *angiogenesis* (blood vessel growth) in triggering AVM formation in mice led to further studies of *antiangiogenesis* drugs in mice and subsequently in humans with severe nose or GI bleeding.[2] These studies are discussed below.

What Causes AVMs to Develop in HHT?

Scientists already know that the genes involved in HHT carry the code, or instructions, for making proteins that control blood vessel growth (angiogenesis); mutations in these genes lead to mistakes in the instructions for these proteins. But the specific mechanisms that result in formation of telangiectasias and AVMs in some, but not all, people with HHT and in some, but not all, parts of the body are not yet known. Nor do we know why different people in the same family (with the same HHT gene) can have AVMs in different organs.

What scientists *have* learned is that *endothelial cells* that form the lining of blood vessels are critical in HHT. The proteins normally made by *ENG* and *ALK1* genes affect the endothelial cells to protect against AVM formation and hemorrhage (in HHT, when those proteins are deficient, AVMs and bleeding are more likely to occur). And scientists now have good evidence that AVM formation depends not only on having a mutation in an HHT gene but also on the presence of *other* genes that influence (or *modify*) the expression of the HHT genes, including variations in the normal, or "good," *ALK1* or *ENG* gene and gene mutations occurring later in life. Various environmental triggers that stimulate new blood vessel growth may also influence the development of AVMs in people with *ALK1* or *ENG* mutations.

The Role of Modifier Genes

A number of researchers have tried to answer the question why HHT symptoms, especially the presence, size, and location of AVMs, vary so much among family members who have the same HHT gene mutation. One explanation is that additional genes interact with the HHT genes to cause the growth of AVMs. These additional genes are called *modifier genes* because they influence how a gene is expressed. Work on identifying modifier genes that affect the expression of HHT genes is ongoing and may lead to improved diagnosis and treatment of HHT. Some studies examine the modifying influence of the *normal ENG* or *ALK1* gene (the one inherited from the non-HHT-affected parent) on the expression of the abnormal, or mutated, *ENG* or *ALK1* gene in people with HHT. Scientists now know that genetic variations in the normal *ENG* gene contribute to the risk of pulmonary AVMs in people with HHT and *ENG* mutations.[3]

Environmental Triggers: Injury, Inflammation, and Macrophages

Studies of knock-out mice led to the idea that *inflammation* (a response to an infection or injury) could be an environmental trigger for AVM development. Mice that were missing *ALK1* developed AVMs in inflamed skin wounds in which *macrophages* (white blood cells that digest bacteria and foreign substances) were present. (This combination of inflammation and an influx of macrophages also occurs in human tissues after injury, trauma, or infection.) When researchers treated the skin wounds with a chemical that kills macrophages (and related cell types), remarkably fewer AVMs formed in the wounds.

In a study under way at the time of this writing, scientists are using genetic models to selectively eliminate macrophages (but not other white blood cells) in the wounds to see if macrophages play an essential role in AVM formation. If this is the case, then drugs targeting macrophages (rather than angiogenesis) might be useful in preventing AVMs in humans.[4] These drugs might have fewer side effects than those that work by inhibiting blood vessel development (see below).

Clinical Research: What Have We Learned So Far?

Clinical research is research done with human beings. Clinical research is used to develop better or safer screening tests, to compare the effectiveness of different drugs or procedures (often after they've been tested in animal models), and to study the effects of behavioral and environmental factors (such as smoking, stress, diet, injury, and so forth) on illness. All these areas are relevant for HHT.

Screening for Lung AVMs: How Can Doctors Get the Most Useful Information in the Safest Way?

You may recall the discussion in chapter 3 of a system for grading the degree of shunting seen on the echo bubble test used to screen for lung AVMs. Years ago, doctors recommended that anyone whose echo bubble test result was positive (showing any degree of shunting) should get a CT scan of the lungs to discover the exact location and size of the AVMs in order to determine whether treatment was needed. It was generally recommended that the CT scan be repeated every five years to see whether the AVMs had grown. But CT scans involve radiation exposure, and many doctors were concerned about repeating this test every five years, especially in children.

Results of a research study using the grading system to compare changes in echo bubble test results and changes on CT scans over the same time periods led to new screening recommendations. In this study, more than 100 patients with negative echo bubble test results (no shunting) were retested after 5, 10, and 15 years. Forty-five percent of patients had a positive test result (developed some degree of shunting) over this time period, but CT scans done at the same time intervals as the echo bubble tests showed that none of the patients developed a *treatable* AVM (all AVMs were tiny). In a second study of 113 patients with a mild degree of shunting, 19 percent developed a moderate degree of shunting over time, but only 6 percent had a treatable AVM identified by a CT scan.

Because the number of treatable AVMs found by CT scans was so low in both the first study group (no shunting on initial screening) and the second (mild shunting on initial screening), many doctors now recommend that *adults* whose initial echo bubble test shows only mild shunting do not need a CT scan right away; instead, they should repeat the echo bubble test in five years and have a CT scan only if they've developed a higher grade of shunting—moderate or severe. Those whose initial echo bubble test result is negative (no shunting) can wait 10–15 years before having a repeat test (to see whether AVMs have developed). This revised screening protocol results in less radiation exposure for many patients and reduced medical expenses, with very little sacrifice in detection of *treatable* AVMs.[5]

Recommendations for lung AVM screening in *children* have also changed as a result of clinical research on the outcomes of embolization. It has been found that children are much more likely than adults to have *reperfusion* (regrowth of abnormal blood vessels) after an embolization. While multiple embolization procedures might eventually be successful in treating the AVM, clinical data suggest that multiple procedures may trigger the growth of new AVMs in children. (One theory is that these procedures create inflammation in the lungs, but this has not been demonstrated with research evidence.) These findings led to the recommendation to delay treating AVMs in children who have no symptoms. Some physicians reason that if treatment of asymptomatic children should be delayed, it makes sense not to perform echo bubble screening in young children. (Others doctors continue to use echo bubble screening, reasoning that if the degree of shunting is severe, early treatment could be beneficial.) Children who *do* have symptoms, such as shortness of breath, low oxygen levels, or difficulty exercising, do need echo bubble screening, which should be followed up with a CT scan if the echo bubble test result is positive. (Children with known or suspected HHT who have not yet been screened for lung AVMs should use prophylactic antibiotics for dental and surgical procedures that could introduce bacteria into the blood.)

Treatment for Lung AVMs: Which Procedure Works Best?

Embolization is usually the best choice for treating lung AVMs. It can be done using either steel coils or a *microvascular* plug (one type is the Amplatzer plug) to block the vessels that supply blood to lung AVMs. While the goal of embolization treatment is to permanently eliminate the AVM, in some cases the blood flows back into the AVM through the coils or plug *after* the embolization; this is called *recanalization*. When this occurs, the AVM must be treated again in order to protect the person from the risk of stroke or brain abscess.

A few recent studies have looked at outcome data on people treated either with plugs or with coils and compared the rates of recanalization for the two types of devices. While there is some evidence for a lower rate of recanalization with plugs, much more research is necessary to determine whether one type of device is truly more effective than the other. Treatment with either coils or plugs will have the best outcomes when done by physicians with expertise in the procedure, most preferably at an HHT Center of Excellence.

Research on the Genes Involved in HHT

As stated in chapter 1, genetic testing for HHT sometimes finds a *variant of uncertain significance (VUS)*. This means that there is a change in the gene, but the change is not clearly associated with HHT. Family members of someone with this result on genetic testing will need to have clinical screening tests to find out whether they have HHT.

Researchers are studying these variants of uncertain significance to try to learn whether these gene changes are found only in family members with a clinical diagnosis of HHT. Families can make it possible for scientists to answer this question by having multiple members (including those who don't have HHT) get genetic testing as part of a research study. Testing is usually provided free when conducted solely for research.

New Drug Treatments to Reduce Bleeding in HHT

In the United States, the Food and Drug Administration (FDA) must approve a drug before doctors can prescribe it or patients can buy it "over the counter." Drugs are approved for specific uses to help guide medical practice. For example, a drug approved to treat viruses should not be used to treat strep throat or other bacterial infections. But it is not illegal or unethical for a doctor to use a drug approved for one illness to treat someone with a different illness if there is some scientific reason to think it might work. Similarly, doctors may use unproven treatments on very ill patients when no other remedy is available. Some doctors write up and publish the results of such experimental treatments; these are called *case reports* or, when several patients were given the treatment, *case series*. *Pilot studies* test new treatments or procedures on a small group of patients to decide whether results warrant launching a bigger study.

While good results from such case reports and pilot studies do not prove that the drug or treatment will work for everyone, these clinical experiments can spark interest in and support for larger *randomized controlled trials* (*RCTs*), which are considered the gold standard in clinical research. In RCTs, patients with similar symptoms or conditions are randomly assigned to different groups, and each group is given a different drug or treatment, usually including a *placebo* (an inactive, or "sugar," pill). The patient does not know which treatment he or she is being given, and in some study designs the researchers do not know either. At the end of the study, the results of the groups are compared to see whether one treatment worked better than the others and, possibly, whether one group showed more negative side effects—or unforeseen benefits—than the others.

Topical Treatments for Nosebleeds

One of the best ways to prevent nosebleeds is to keep the nose moist. There are numerous sprays, oils, and ointments that people apply to the inside of the nostrils to help reduce nosebleeds. Some, such as petroleum jelly, are known to act simply as a barrier to dryness, but others, such as estrogen creams, were thought to have a direct effect on the development of telangiectasias in the nose. Recently the drug *Avastin* (bevacizumab) has been explored as a treatment for bleeding in HHT. Avastin, which is approved for treatment of some cancers, works by reducing the blood supply to tumors. Many were hopeful that Avastin used as a nose spray would reduce nosebleeds. A topical treatment for nosebleeds that really works would be a boon to many people with HHT.

In the North American Study of Epistaxis (NOSE), an RCT of topical treatments for nosebleeds, 121 patients with moderate to severe nosebleeds used a nose spray for 12 weeks. Researchers compared the effects of three different sprays that might have direct effects on bleeding: Avastin, *tranexamic acid* (a drug that promotes clotting), and *estriol* (low-dose estrogen); saline spray was used as the placebo. To measure whether nosebleeds improved with treatment, researchers compared Epistaxis Severity Scores (described in chapter 2) and nosebleed frequency before and after treatment.

The NOSE study showed that for nosebleed frequency there was no more benefit from Avastin or tranexamic acid than from saline (placebo) and that estriol actually led to *worse* outcomes than saline. Possibly the dose of medications was too low to be effective, or perhaps topical application is not an effective way to use these drugs.[6] Perhaps a gel would have been more effective than a spray. Clearing or irrigating the nose prior to use of the spray, which was not done in this study, might have improved the effectiveness of the medications. These ideas may be tested in future research. (Some patients report that using estrogen cream, rather than spray, in the nose reduces nosebleeds, but this has not been studied in a research trial.)

Topical treatment is not the only route for medications to reduce bleeding. In clinical practice and in many research studies drugs are given orally, intravenously, or by direct injection into abnormal blood vessels. Recently, much of the research on drugs to reduce bleeding has focused on

Avastin and other drugs that inhibit blood vessel growth (antiangiogenesis or anti-VEGF drugs).

Anti-VEGF Drugs

As noted earlier, the endothelial cells that line the blood vessels are critical in HHT. *Vascular endothelial growth factor (VEGF)* is a protein that promotes angiogenesis (blood vessel growth) and influences the development of both normal and abnormal blood vessels by acting on endothelial cells. VEGF is found in higher than normal amounts in the blood of people with HHT. It's possible that excess VEGF causes telangiectasias and AVMs to develop and makes these abnormal vessels more prone to bleeding. Drugs that block the action of VEGF (anti-VEGF or antiangiogenesis drugs) may reduce blood vessel growth and/or bleeding from abnormal vessels. Avastin is one anti-VEGF drug that's been used in a number of small studies to treat nosebleeds and GI bleeding, and some larger studies are now under way.

As the NOSE study demonstrated, Avastin used as a nose spray was no more effective than saline. But a small study comparing patients with heavy nosebleeds using either laser treatment alone or laser treatment combined with *injections* of Avastin inside the nose found that those who received the Avastin injections had fewer nosebleeds, needed fewer blood transfusions, and reported improved quality of life.[7] Because this study was small and lacked a control (placebo or alternate treatment) group, it could not show definitively that Avastin injections were effective for a majority of patients. Also, about 40 percent of the patients in this study developed a hole in the nasal septum, a serious adverse side effect of treatment. Recent modifications of the injection technique have reduced the likelihood of this complication in patients treated since that study was conducted. But because its effectiveness and safety have not been proven, most physicians recommend Avastin injections only for patients who continue to have serious nosebleeds and need blood transfusions despite other treatments. A new RCT of Avastin will be useful in deciding whether to use these injections in patients with a wider range of nosebleed severity (see below).

Several research studies in the United States and Europe (including more than 50 patients altogether) have demonstrated benefits of Avastin given *intravenously* as a treatment for severe nosebleeds.[8] Thus far, there has been no controlled study of a large group of patients demonstrating the benefits and risks of this treatment.

GI bleeding from telangiectasias sometimes worsens as people age, resulting in anemia and dependence on blood transfusions. Several case studies have used Avastin given intravenously to one or a few patients with serious GI bleeding. They report increased hemoglobin levels (that is, improved anemia), a reduced need for blood transfusions, and fewer visits to the ER or hospital during the year following treatment. At this time, there is no larger study that demonstrates Avastin's effectiveness in treating GI bleeding.

Other Drugs to Reduce Nosebleeds

Tamoxifen is a drug used to treat breast cancer by reducing the action of estrogen in breast tissue. But in blood vessels (and some other tissues) tamoxifen actually *increases* the action of estrogen. Tamoxifen was studied as a treatment for nosebleeds in 25 patients with HHT, who were randomly assigned to be treated with oral tamoxifen or a placebo for six months. The group treated with tamoxifen had less frequent and less severe nosebleeds, and some showed improved hemoglobin.[9] Tamoxifen is currently used in some clinical settings for treatment of nosebleeds.

Tranexamic acid is a drug that promotes blood clotting. While not effective as a topical treatment in the NOSE study, tranexamic acid given orally in a multicenter European RCT with more than 100 patients[10] and in a smaller RCT in Germany[11] resulted in a moderate reduction in the duration and number of nosebleeds. Further studies are needed to confirm the safety of tranexamic acid and determine which patients are most likely to benefit from it. However, these studies provided support for the effectiveness of tranexamic acid, which is currently used in clinical settings for nonsurgical treatment of moderate to severe nosebleeds. (Because it promotes clotting, tranexamic acid should *not* be used for people who are at risk for blood clots.)

Bazedoxifene, another drug that facilitates the effects of estrogen and is used to treat osteoporosis, shows potential for treatment of bleeding in HHT. In a pilot study of five women with HHT its use resulted in decreased frequency and severity of nosebleeds (and decreased levels of VEGF following treatment).[12] More research on this drug is needed before it can be recommended as a routine treatment for bleeding in HHT.

HHT and Other Health Outcomes

HHT and Life Expectancy

Some researchers have raised questions about how HHT affects overall life expectancy and what effects HHT might have on other health outcomes. A questionnaire study that asked people who were in the databases of two HHT Centers of Excellence about their parents' age at death provide evidence that HHT plays a role in shortening the life span of people who are not screened and treated for lung and brain AVMs.[13] Ninety-five percent of the parents had not been screened for lung or brain AVMs prior to their death, and while parents with the *ALK1* mutation had normal life expectancies, those with endoglin mutations died about seven years earlier on average than the parents without HHT. *Women* with endoglin mutations were most at risk for earlier death because of complications from HHT. This study highlights the importance of screening HHT patients for organ involvement.

HHT and Cancer Survival

While endoglin mutations may lead to more complications than *ALK1* mutations in people with HHT who have not been properly screened for organ involvement, endoglin mutations may have a role in *improving* survival rates for some illnesses, such as cancer. A group of researchers did a retrospective study to look at the survival rates for various types of cancer in people with HHT (who are expected to have reduced levels of endoglin in their blood). Comparing survival rates of people with cancer but without HHT with the survival rates of people with cancer and with HHT, they found that survival rates were improved for the people *with* HHT. The survival rates in women with HHT and breast cancer were better than those in women without HHT who had breast cancer.[14] This finding opens the door to further research on the role of endoglin in cancer and to studies of how HHT affects survival in people with other chronic illnesses.

HHT and Myocardial Infarction

An international survey study of more than 1,000 people with HHT found another potentially protective effect of HHT: reported rates of myocardial infarction (heart attack) were *less* in the HHT group than in the general population. The rates of reported heart attacks for people whose parents and grandparents had been diagnosed with HHT were also lower, especially for men.[15]

HHT and Quality of Life

As discussed in part II, HHT affects emotions, relationships, and work and leisure activities—in other words, quality of life. This is an area where research is limited, but several studies in Germany, Norway, and the United States have found that quality of life is related to the severity of HHT symptoms and to some extent to the coping skills that people use to handle stress. In particular, nosebleed severity and time spent caring for nosebleeds are linked to more stress, anxiety, and sadness; bleeding and other HHT symptoms that interfere with work, athletic activities, or other daily routines are most likely to cause distress. General debility, fatigue, and weakness owing to liver involvement in HHT also have a negative impact on quality of life.

A recent study examining the life experiences of 19 people with HHT revealed that many were concerned about other family members' health and worried about developing more symptoms as they got older. Despite feelings of frustration, embarrassment, worry, and sadness, people also described acceptance of HHT and adjustment to its impact on their lives, including strategies to manage the social impact of nosebleeds, and taking steps to protect their health as much as possible. Finally, this study looked at how people tell others in their lives about HHT. At work, disclosure of HHT was most often made on a "need to know" basis, such as telling an immediate superior if nosebleeds would require frequent trips to the restroom. Friends or dating partners were usually told about HHT as the relationship became closer or more "serious." People with HHT found it easier than did people with some other genetic diseases to tell others about their illness, maybe because nosebleeds made it obvious that something was wrong and they often felt the need to give others an explanation.[16]

Further studies of the emotional experiences of people with HHT may encourage doctors to pay attention not only to the medical consequences of HHT but to the emotional and social consequences as well and to help counselors and psychologists better understand the specific types of supports and coping strategies that can improve adjustment and quality of life for people with HHT.

The Cutting Edge: New and Ongoing Clinical Research Studies

At the time of this writing, several new pilot studies and RCTs are in progress or are recruiting subjects. Building on the results of earlier case reports or small studies, these new research projects aim to demonstrate more definitively that a particular drug is effective in treating an HHT symptom and/or to determine the safety of a new drug or treatment.

Studies of Drugs to Reduce Bleeding
Bevacizumab (Avastin)

An RCT of bevacizumab (Avastin) in the treatment of nosebleeds funded by Cure HHT and the American Academy of Otolaryngology is currently under way at the Stanford School of Medicine. It will compare the effectiveness of bevacizumab injection with that of saline (placebo) injection combined with electrocautery for treating HHT-related nosebleeds. Patients in the study will receive the injections while they are anesthetized for electrocautery surgery. Based on earlier studies with this drug, researchers are hopeful that bevacizumab injections will be shown to reduce the frequency and severity of nosebleeds, improve quality of life, and reduce medical costs more effectively than the placebo. Patients can enroll in this study on the Cure HHT website at http://curehht .org/2015/11/a-randomized-controlled-trial-of-bevacizumab-for-hht -related-epistaxis/.

Pomalidomide

Pomalidomide, another drug with antiangiogenesis effects, is currently used in the treatment of multiple myeloma (bone marrow cancer). A new research study is being conducted at the Cleveland Clinic to look at the effects of pomalidomide on people with HHT who need ongoing blood transfusions or iron infusions because of severe GI bleeding or nosebleeds. Researchers hope that the drug will decrease the need for blood transfusions by 50 percent. Patients can enroll in this study on the Cure

HHT website at http://curehht.org/2015/11/pomalidomide-in-hht-and
-transfusion-dependent-vascular-ectasia-a-phase-i-study/.

Pazopanib

Pazopanib is a chemotherapy drug used to treat renal cancer. Because of
its antiangiogenesis effects, this drug is currently being considered for treatment of bleeding in HHT. In a small study, pazopanib was beneficial, but
further studies were discontinued when the drug was sold to another pharmaceutical company. Cure HHT and the researchers are currently in talks
with the new company, advocating for continuation of this promising work.
For updated information on this study and when you might be able to enroll as a subject, visit https://clinicaltrials.gov/ct2/show/NCT02204371
?term=hht&rank=39.

Timolol

Timolol is a medicine commonly used to treat high blood pressure and glaucoma. Because it narrows blood vessels and reduces the amount of blood
flowing through them, timolol may reduce nasal telangiectasias and bleeding. Researchers in France are now recruiting subjects to study the effect
of a timolol nose spray on nosebleed severity, anemia, blood transfusions,
and quality of life in people with moderate to severe nosebleeds. There is
currently no research trial of timolol for nosebleeds in the United States.

    As yet, there is no research study comparing the effectiveness of these
different medications and it is not clear which medications are most appropriate for individuals with varying degrees of bleeding or different genetic mutations. Future research will be useful in guiding doctors to choose
the best medication for each individual with HHT-related bleeding.

Studies of Drugs to Reduce Skin Telangiectasias

Timolol, described above as a treatment for high blood pressure, glaucoma,
and possibly nosebleeds, has also been used successfully to treat skin *hemangiomas,* red "birthmarks" that can have an unpleasant appearance on the
face. Timolol limits the blood flow to the hemangiomas by narrowing blood
vessels; the same mechanism might work in reducing blood flow to skin
telangiectasias. Researchers in the Johns Hopkins Department of Derma-
tology are now conducting a pilot study of timolol to treat telangiectasias

on the skin in people with HHT. You can find more information about how to participate in this study at http://curehht.org/?s=tim. Another study on timolol for treating telangiectasias is being conducted at St. Michael's Hospital in Toronto, affiliated with the University of Toronto; more information is available at https://clinicaltrials.gov/ct2/show/NCT01752049.

The Brain AVM Study

As discussed in chapter 3, brain AVMs are easy to find, but it's much less clear how to manage them. That's because scientists don't fully understand what makes brain AVMs bleed. Before people with HHT were routinely screened for brain AVMs, most patients didn't know they had a brain AVM unless it caused symptoms such as seizures or hemorrhaging. While much can be learned by looking back at the medical and life histories of patients after they have a bleed, the best way to learn about risk factors is to track patients with known brain AVMs and observe what happens to them as time goes by. The Brain AVM Study, led by Michael Lawton, MD, and Marie Faughnan, MD, is doing just that.

Officially titled "Cerebral Hemorrhage Risk in Hereditary Hemorrhagic Telangiectasia (HHT)," the study does not change the clinical monitoring and treatment of HHT patients who enroll in the study—this will be done by their own doctors—but it keeps track of their progress, symptoms, treatments, and how they do after treatment. By collecting medical data (clinical, laboratory, and imaging data and blood samples) on participating patients at regular intervals, the study aims to determine the genetic and clinical factors that result in a high risk for bleeding from brain AVMs in people with HHT. These data will help guide decisions about how to treat brain AVMs in individual patients with various risk factors and will promote research on new methods of treating brain AVMs.

Data for people with HHT and people with two other rare diseases that cause brain AVMs are being collected by scientists in the Brain Vascular Malformation Consortium (BVMC). The BVMC is a part of the National Institutes of Health (NIH) Rare Disease Clinical Research Network (RDCRN), which is funding this research. HHT Centers of Excellence across North America are now actively recruiting HHT patients to participate in this study. If you are interested in participating, contact your local HHT Center of Excellence (see the "Resources" section of this book) or Cure HHT.

Our HHT Registry: Outcomes Research for HHT

Plans are currently under way to launch an HHT registry to promote research on outcomes. A medical research *registry* is an organized system that collects data on patients with a specific medical condition over time. The registry observes but does not interfere with patients' symptoms and outcomes over the course of their disease, including any treatments they have along the way. Like the Brain AVM Study, the HHT outcomes registry would not change the medical care of any individual HHT patient. The aim of the registry is to generate new knowledge about many facets of HHT in order to guide future research and ultimately create better treatments for all HHT patients. The registry is very important for advancing research on HHT. Access to this type of patient registry may be a determining factor in pharmaceutical companies' decision whether to invest in drug development for HHT.

The registry, known as Our HHT Registry: Outcomes Research for HHT, will track clinical data (symptoms, family history, risk factors), radiographic tests (x-ray, CT scan, MRI scan), genetic data, and treatment information covering every aspect of HHT. As with any research, patients will be included in the registry only if they voluntarily consent to participate, and their identities will not be available to those using the registry for research.

The registry will focus on the *outcomes* of people with HHT (severity of symptoms, quality of life, heart failure, stroke, severe bleeding, and death), the personal factors that affect these outcomes (genetics, lifestyle, age, sex, and so forth), and the therapies used by patients. The information gathered in the registry can be used to plan and target clinical research studies of new drugs and other treatments.

Cure HHT awarded the Geisel School of Medicine at Dartmouth a $131,000 grant to develop the initial database for the outcomes registry. A pilot study of the registry system with two HHT Centers of Excellence is the next step. Ultimately, the registry will link all North American HHT Centers of Excellence, potentially including a much greater number of patients than could be studied at any one center or hospital. However, the registry project is very expensive, and future progress will depend on the availability of funding. Raising money for the registry project is one of Cure HHT's strategic priorities.

How Research Is Funded

There are several main sources for funding research projects in the United States. The biggest source of funding for basic science research is grants awarded to scientists based on competitive applications, most of which come from the National Institutes of Health or other government agencies concerned with health, medicine, and science. The NIH funds clinical studies too, but drug companies provide much of the funding for research on development of new drugs or on the use of existing drugs for new purposes. Some companies that manufacture medical devices, such as coils, catheters, or scanners, fund research related to the use of these devices. Many smaller grants are awarded by private research foundations, community hospitals, or universities. And some funds come from patient-funded foundations or organizations concerned with a particular disease. Cure HHT, with donations from its members and other individual donors, has been able to give small start-up grants to a number of promising researchers. In several cases, the projects yielded exciting results and the funded scientists subsequently applied for and received much larger NIH grants to continue their research.

Because the grant application process is competitive, funds are limited, and priority is given to serious disorders that affect a large percentage of the US population (such as heart disease and cancer), government funds for rare diseases like HHT are sparse. Cure HHT and many of its members support legislative efforts to pass the HHT Data Act (discussed in chapter 6), which would increase federal funds for HHT research. Several big pharmaceutical companies have shown some interest in funding research on treatments for HHT, and this may become a bigger source of funds in the future. But in the meantime, grass-roots funding of Cure HHT is an essential source of support for HHT research. If you are interested in supporting research on HHT by making a donation or organizing a fundraising event, contact Cure HHT at www.curehht.org. This is one way that you can personally contribute to finding better treatments for HHT.

Becoming a Research Subject

You may have felt excited the last time you read a headline or tweet reporting that research showed that a new drug reduced bleeding in HHT. Maybe you even called your doctor to ask whether you could get the new drug as soon as possible. But did you ever wonder who made it possible for the scientists to find out that the new drug works? The answer is people like you. Another way you can contribute to the discovery of new treatments for HHT is to participate in research by enrolling in the Brain AVM Study, by participating in a survey study, or by becoming a subject in a clinical trial.

It is through clinical research that scientists answer questions about HHT—everything from what's the most effective drug for bleeding to how HHT affects emotional adjustment to when brain AVMs should be treated. The answers might require a pilot study or an RCT, an interview or a patient survey, or collecting patients' medical data in a registry or database. What all these studies have in common is that they depend on *volunteers*— real people with HHT—who are willing to take a new drug without knowing that it's going to work (or even whether they are taking the real drug or a placebo); to share their medical and genetic histories; and to honestly answer questions about their medical and/or emotional symptoms. Without the help of volunteer research subjects like you and me, progress toward developing new HHT treatments would come to a screeching halt.

Why Participate?

Participating in research as a subject is a *choice*; certainly it is not a requirement for getting good medical care. But there are some very good reasons to think about participating in HHT research:

The research study could be personally beneficial to you. For example, if you need regular blood transfusions, you might benefit from being part of a study on a new treatment to reduce bleeding. If you are embarrassed by telangiectasias on your face, your participation in a drug study might be a good opportunity to get rid of those troubling red spots. Being part of a study is sometimes the only way to get a new drug that is not yet approved for use by the FDA (or an equivalent agency, if you live outside the United States). Additionally, most studies provide the experimental drug for free, so you don't have to pay for it or worry about insurance coverage. Most research studies will also reimburse you for travel expenses, and some studies will even pay you for participating.

The research study could benefit your family. Even if you are less likely to benefit personally from being in a particular study, your participation in HHT research might contribute to finding effective treatments that will one day help your own children, grandchildren, or great-grandchildren, maybe even save their lives.

Participating in research promotes scientific knowledge that potentially benefits all people. Being a subject in HHT research advances knowledge of HHT. Through better understanding of blood vessel development, genetic mutations, and many medical symptoms shared by HHT and other diseases, the research has the potential to benefit people with a wide variety of health conditions.

Who Can Participate?

Some research studies have specific eligibility requirements, for example, having had at least four blood transfusions in the past year or having had a moderate to high Epistaxis Severity Score. This is often the case, because a certain degree of symptom severity is necessary to accurately test whether the research drug is effective in reducing symptoms or because potential side effects of the drug, even if they are very mild, outweigh the potential benefits for those whose symptoms are minimal. (For example, someone with occasional, mild nosebleeds would be advised to use topical moisturizers in their nose rather than take an experimental drug for bleeding that could cause nausea and weight loss.)

While you may not be eligible to participate in every research study, some research studies are open to anyone with HHT. These include surveys, studies based on information contained in patient registries, and studies of drugs with minimal or no known side effects. Participation in this type of research, in which there is virtually no risk to your health, is a way to help others with HHT and perhaps contribute to knowledge that will be helpful to you personally at some point in the future.

Is It Safe to Be a Research Subject?

When you participate in a research study that involves taking a drug, having an injection, or some other medical intervention, you are protected from harm to the greatest extent possible. If your symptoms don't get better (because the drug doesn't work or you got the placebo) or if you get worse, you have the right to leave the study (or the researcher may request that you leave for your own safety) and try a different type of treatment. Research studies are designed to minimize and carefully monitor participants for potential side effects; if you experience any side effects, the study doctors are responsible for treating you. You may be able to tolerate mild side effects, or you may have to discontinue participation.

Research done at accredited medical institutions or funded by the NIH, other scientific granting agencies, and drug companies must be approved by an institutional review board (IRB). An IRB is made up of clinicians and scientists with a range of expertise, doctors or scientists who specialize in the particular area being studied, health consumers, and experts in medical ethics. Its job is to ensure that the research is conducted safely and ethically and protects human subjects. The IRB requires, among other things, that subjects be thoroughly informed of the risks and benefits of the research and alternatives to participation; that treatment be provided in the event that participation in the study causes medical harm; and that the amount of risk subjects are exposed to is minimized.

When you join a clinical study, you should be given an informed consent document that outlines the purpose, risks, and potential benefits of the study; payment, if any, for participating; and information on whom to contact if you feel you have been harmed in any way. This document should contain an official stamp of approval from the IRB. You should also be given an opportunity to ask any and all questions about the study before you consent to participate. When you sign the consent form, you should be given a copy. *Remember*: you can never be forced to participate in a study, and if you change your mind, you have the option of withdrawing your consent and leaving the study at any time for any reason.

Where Can I Find a Study?

Most clinical research studies about HHT are posted on the Cure HHT website and on the websites of the HHT Centers of Excellence or other medical institutions conducting the research. Many research studies are conducted at multiple locations simultaneously, in order to have enough participants. Your doctor might tell you about research studies on your particular symptoms or problems. You can also visit www.clinicaltrials.gov, a registry and results database of publicly and privately supported clinical studies conducted around the world. If you search for "hereditary hemorrhagic telangiectasia" (you have to spell it out; don't use "HHT" as your search term) on that website, you can find studies that are currently recruiting subjects with HHT. You can also see which studies are in progress, as well as the results of completed studies. If you would like to be a subject in a clinical study of a medication, surgery, or procedure, it's a good idea to check with your HHT doctor and/or primary care physician before enrolling.

On the Horizon: Gene Therapy

Gene therapy is an experimental therapy that uses changes in genes to treat or prevent disease. Although it may eventually be an effective treatment for many diseases, including genetic disorders like HHT, gene therapy has many risks, and more studies are needed to make sure it can be done safely. At this time, gene therapy is used only in clinical research trials and only for serious illnesses for which there is no other treatment.

The main approaches to gene therapy include inactivating a mutated gene; replacing a mutated gene with a healthy copy of the gene; or introducing a new gene into the body to help fight a disease. HHT researchers are using animal models to investigate how genes can be altered to improve blood vessel development and prevent AVMs from developing and how to enhance the function of the "good" copy of a person's HHT gene—or other modifier genes—so it will compensate for the faulty "instructions" of the mutated copy. This type of research in animals could eventually pave the way for development of a gene therapy for humans with HHT.

The Future of HHT

The future looks promising for people with HHT. Advances in diagnosis, screening, treatment, and prevention have made HHT a much more manageable disease in 2017 than it was for previous generations. The availability of genetic testing and increases in public awareness and physician training are likely to improve the diagnosis rate for HHT considerably. With proper diagnosis and education, most people with HHT can live a good life.

For people with more disabling consequence of bleeding from HHT, the current flurry of research on medications to reduce bleeding is likely to identify more effective treatments in the near future. There have been refinements in procedures, such as laser cautery techniques, surgical approaches, and treatments for AVMs, and these are likely to continue, producing better outcomes.

Medical care for people with HHT is increasingly available as the number of HHT Centers of Excellence continues to grow. Children can be screened early in life for HHT, and people with HHT have access to more knowledge about how to care for and manage their children's HHT symptoms.

Finally, there is more social and emotional support for people with HHT than ever before. Many people with HHT feel freer than ever to talk about their illness and how it affects their lives and more empowered to manage their HHT, spread awareness, and advocate for themselves and others with HHT. Social media have brought support into people's living rooms, while patient and family conferences and local support groups provide the opportunity for face-to-face support and sharing.

All of us with HHT hope for a cure in our lifetime. And medical research is taking us in that direction. But we don't have to wait for a cure to start living a better life with HHT. Right now, starting today, we can improve our health and quality of life by staying informed, seeking expert medical care, and learning how to manage our symptoms. And most importantly, we can have compassion for ourselves and support one another in our struggles and triumphs with HHT.

Notes

Chapter 3. HHT's Hidden Dangers

1. The material on lung AVMs in this chapter was improved by input from Daniel Picus, MD, professor of radiology and surgery, chief of the Division of Diagnostic Radiology and an interventional radiology consultant for the HHT Center of Excellence at Washington University School of Medicine in St. Louis, Missouri. The material on brain AVMs was improved by input from Karel terBrugge, MD, FRCPC, the David Braley and Nancy Gordon Chair in Interventional Neuroradiology, professor of radiology and surgery and head of the Division of Neuroradiology and member of the HHT Center of Excellence at the University of Toronto in Ontario, Canada.

2. Quoted in "Living with PH and HHT, a patient's experience," by Christine Fini, in *Pathlight*, the newsletter of the Pulmonary Hypertension Association, www.PHAssociation.org, 2010.

Chapter 4. Taking Care of Yourself

1. Quoted in "Life Experiences of Individuals with Hereditary Hemorrhagic Telangiectasia and Disclosing Outside the Family: A Qualitative Analysis," by L. A. Higa, J. McDonald, D. O. Himes, and E. Rothwell, *Journal of Community Genetics* 7 (2016): 84.

Chapter 7. Frontiers in HHT Research

1. Quoted from an interview on the Cure HHT website, http://curehht.org /2016/07/hht-research-its-in-the-genes/.

2. S. Tual-Chalot, S. P. Oh, and H. M. Arthur, "Mouse Models of Hereditary Hemorrhagic Telangiectasia: Recent Advances and Future Challenges," *Frontiers in Genetics* 6 (2015): 25.

3. T. G. Letteboer, M. Benzinou, C. B. Merrick, D. A. Quigley, K. Zhau, I. Kim, M. D. To, D. M. Jablons, J. K. P. van Amstel, C. J. J. Westermann, S. Dupuis-Girod, G. Lesca, J. H. Berg, A. Balmain, and R. J. Akhurst, "Genetic Variation in the Functional *ENG* Allele Inherited from the Non-affected Parent Associates with Presence of Pulmonary Arteriovenous Malformation in

Hereditary Hemorrhagic Telangiectasia 1 (HHT1) and May Influence Expression of PTPN14," *Frontiers in Genetics* 6 (2015): 67.

4. S. P. Oh, "Macrophages Are Essential for the Formation of AVM's in HHT patients," summary of research hypothesis under study funded by a National Institutes of Health RO1 grant, announced on the Cure HHT website, Apr 13, 2016. Dr. Oh's preliminary research on this topic, "The Role of Macrophages in the Pathogenesis of HHT," was funded by a seed grant from Cure HHT.

5. S. Velthuis, E. Buscarini, J. R. Gossage, R. J. Snijder, J. J. Mager, and M. C. Post, "Clinical Implications of Pulmonary Shunting on Saline Contrast Echocardiography," *Journal of the American Society of Echocardiography* 28, no. 3 (2015): 255–63.

6. K. J. Whitehead, N. B. Sautter, J. P. McWilliams, M. M. Chakinala, C. A. Merlo, M. H. Johnson, M. James, E. M. Everett, M. S. Clancy, M. E. Faughnan, S. P. Oh, S. E. Olitsky, R. E. Pyeritz, and J. R. Gossage, "Effect of Topical Intranasal Therapy on Epistaxis Frequency in Patients with Hereditary Hemorrhagic Telangiectasia: A Randomized Clinical Trial," *Journal of the American Medical Society* 316, no. 9 (2016): 943–51.

7. J. Simonds, F. Miller, J. Mandel, and T. M. Davidson, "The Effect of Bevacizumab (Avastin) Treatment on Epistaxis in Hereditary Hemorrhagic Telangiectasia," *Laryngoscope* 119, no. 5 (2009): 988–92.

8. H. Arthur, U. Geisthoff, J. R. Gossage, C. C. W. Hughes, P. Lacombe, M. E. Meek, P. Oh, B. L. Roman, S. O. Trerotola, S. Velthuis, and W. Wooderchak-Donahue, "Executive Summary of the 11th HHT International Scientific Conference," *Angiogenesis* 18 (2015): 511–24.

9. E. Yaniv, M. Preis, T. Hadar, J. Shrevo, and M. Haddad, "Antiestrogen Therapy for Hereditary Hemorrhagic Telangiectasia: A Double-blind Placebo-controlled Clinical Trial," *Laryngoscope* 119 (2009): 284–88.

10. S. Gaillard, S. Dupuis-Girod, F. Boutitie, S. Riviere, S. Moriniere, P.-Y. Hatron, G. Manfredi, P. Kaminsky, A.-L. Capitaine, P. Roy, F. Gueyffier, and H. Plauchu, for the ATERO Study Group, "Tranexamic Acid for Epistaxis in Hereditary Hemorrhagic Telangiectasia Patients: A European Cross-over Controlled Trial in a Rare Disease," *Journal of Thrombosis and Haemostasis* 12 (2014): 1494–1502.

11. U. W. Geisthoff, U. T. Seyfert, M. Kubler, B. Bieg, P. K. Plinkert, and J. Konig, "Treatment of Epistaxis in Hereditary Hemorrhagic Telangiectasia with Tranexamic Acid—A Double Blind Placebo Controlled Cross-over Phase IIIB Study," *Thrombosis Research* 134 (2014): 565–71.

12. R. Zarrabeitia, L. Ojeda-Fernandez, L. Recio, C. Bernabeu, J. A. Parra, and V. Albinana, "Bazedoxifene, a New Orphan Drug for the Treatment of Bleeding in Hereditary Haemorrhagic Telangiectasia," *Thrombosis and Haemostatis* 115, no. 6 (2016): 1081–1248.

13. E. M. deGussem, C. P. Edwards, A. E. Hosman, C. J. Westermann, R. J. Snijder, M. E. Faughnan, and J. J. Mager, "Life Expectancy of Parents with Hereditary Hemorrhagic Telangiectasia," *Orphanet Journal of Rare Diseases* 11 (April 2016): 46.

14. C. W. Duarte, K. Murray, F. L. Lucas, K. Fairfield, H. Miller, P. Brooks, and C. P. Vary, "Improved Survival Outcomes in Cancer Patients with Hereditary Hemorrhagic Telangiectasia," *Cancer Epidemiology, Biomarkers and Prevention* 23, no. 1 (January 2014): 117–25.

15. C. L. Shovlin, I. Awan, Z. Cahilog, F. N. Abdulla, and A. E. Guttmacher, "Reported Cardiac Phenotypes in Hereditary Hemorrhagic Telangiectasis Emphasize Burdens from Arrhythmias, Anemia and Its Treatments, but Suggest Reduced Rates of Myocardial Infarction," *International Journal of Cardiology* 215 (July 2016): 179–85.

16. L. A. Higa, J. McDonald, D. O. Himes, and E. Rothwell, "Life Experiences of Individuals with Hereditary Hemorrhagic Telangiectasia and Disclosing outside the Family: A Qualitative Analysis," *Journal of Community Genetics* 7 (2016): 81–89.

Glossary

abscess. An infected, inflamed area in the body where pus collects.

ACVRL1. See *ALK1.*

ALK1. One of the genes known to cause HHT.

Amicar. Trade name for tranexamic acid, a drug that promotes blood clotting.

anemia. A condition caused by not having enough hemoglobin or red blood cells, often resulting from chronic or severe bleeding and causing weakness, fatigue, or shortness of breath.

aneurysm. A weakened and enlarged area of a blood vessel that is prone to bleeding.

angiogenesis. Blood vessel growth or development.

angiogram. A test or procedure used to examine or treat blood vessels of an organ such as the brain or lung. A small tube (catheter) is inserted into a vein or artery. A dye is then injected, which allows all the blood vessels to be seen with high-speed x-ray pictures.

animal model. An animal in which scientists create diseases or genetic changes that mimic those in humans in order to study the diseases and the effects of medications and procedures before testing them on humans.

arrhythmia. An abnormal heart rhythm (beat).

arterial blood gas (ABG) test. A test in which blood is taken from an artery to measure the oxygen and/or carbon dioxide levels.

arteriogram. See **angiogram.**

arteriovenous malformation (AVM). An abnormal, direct connection between an artery and a vein in which capillaries are missing.

ascites. Swelling of the abdominal cavity owing to an abnormal accumulation of fluid that can be caused by liver failure.

asymptomatic. Having no obvious symptoms.

autosomal dominant. A genetic term describing a condition or characteristic that affects men and women equally and has a 50 percent chance of being passed on to each child of the affected parent.

Avastin. Trade name for bevacizumab, a drug that inhibits blood vessel growth.

AVM. See **Arteriovenous malformation.**

bevacizumab. See **Avastin.**

bilateral. On or affecting both sides of the body, for example, both arms or both sides of the face.

biliary ischemia. Lack of oxygen to the bile ducts, causing damage to the ducts and contributing to liver failure. It can be caused by symptomatic liver AVMs.

biopsy. Removal of a small piece of body tissue for microscopic examination, to test for cancer or other abnormalities.

bipolar electrocautery. A technique that can be used to treat nasal telangiectasias in which electricity is passed through the tissue to heat (cauterize) it.

bubble echo test. See **echo bubble test**.

capillaries. The smallest blood vessels, where blood is normally transmittetd from arteries to veins. Capillaries filter the blood in the lungs, preventing debris from going to the brain and body.

catheter. A small plastic tube that is inserted into a vein or elsewhere in the body. In HHT, catheters are used most commonly to repair lung AVMs. See **embolization**.

CAT scan (computed axial tomography). An x-ray test that uses computer reconstruction of multiple images of an organ to diagnose a stroke, AVM, brain abscess, or other condition.

cautery. Use of heat to stop bleeding or destroy tissues; it can be used with nasal telangiectasias to control bleeding in HHT.

CBC (complete blood count). A standard panel of blood tests that includes tests for hemoglobin levels and hematocrit (percentage of blood volume made up of red blood cells).

cerebral. Related to the brain, e.g., a cerebral AVM.

chemical cautery. Cauterization technique using silver nitrate to destroy telangiectasias.

chromosomes. Microscopic particles within the cells of the body that contain genes. Genes for HHT are located on chromosomes 9 and 12 and at least one other chromosome. See **genes**.

clinical depression. A mental health condition marked by sad mood, sleep and appetite changes, hopelessness, excessive guilt, difficulty concentrating, and suicidal thoughts.

coblation. See **cold ablation**.

coil embolization. See **embolization**.

cold ablation. A procedure for removing nasal telangiectasias using radiofrequency energy and saline that causes minimal injury to surrounding healthy tissue.

congenital. A condition that is present from the time of birth but not necessarily hereditary.

Curaçao criteria. The diagnostic criteria for HHT established in 1999 by the Scientific Advisory Board of the HHT Foundation International, Inc.

Cure HHT. The nonprofit organization dedicated to HHT awareness, education, support, and research, previously named HHT Foundation International.

cyanotic. The bluish color of the skin when the lungs are unable to provide enough oxygen to the blood.

depression. See **clinical depression.**

diagnosis. The process of identifying a disease based on symptoms, medical history, and family history.

diffuse. Spread out widely, not concentrated; for example, diffuse lung AVMs are scattered throughout the lungs.

DNA. The basic chemical building blocks of genes.

echo bubble test. A test to detect AVMs in the lung. A sterile solution that has been shaken to create microbubbles is injected into a vein in the arm, and ultrasound images of the heart are recorded to track the movement of the bubbles.

echocardiogram. A test that looks at the function of the heart using images generated by ultrasound waves. Echocardiograms can be used to diagnose heart defects and pulmonary hypertension.

electrocautery. A technique in which electric current is passed through tissue to heat (cauterize) and destroy it.

embolism. Blockage of a blood vessel, usually by a blood clot, as in embolic stroke.

embolization. A treatment for an AVM in which a catheter is used to place a device or substance in a blood vessel to block off the blood flow to an AVM.

embolotherapy. See **embolization.**

endoglin (ENG). One of the genes known to cause HHT.

endoscopy. Examination or treatment of the gastrointestinal tract (esophagus, stomach, small intestine, and colon) using a small tube inserted in the mouth or rectum.

endothelium. The layer of cells that lines the blood vessels.

ENT. A doctor who specializes in the ears, nose, and throat. Many people with HHT see an ENT for treatment of nosebleeds.

epistaxis. The medical term for nosebleeds.

estrogen. The primary female sex hormone. It may play a role in blood vessel growth.

fistula. An abnormal opening or connection between two organs or blood vessels.

gadolinium. A type of dye (contrast) used in MRI screening for brain AVMs.

gastroenterologist (GI). A doctor who treats diseases of the gastrointestinal tract (esophagus, stomach, small intestine, and colon).

gene. The linear sequence of chemicals on a segment of DNA that provides the coded instructions for particular proteins and leads to the expression and transmission of inherited traits. See also **hereditary.**

gene therapy. A therapy that involves inserting corrective genes into the genetic material of a patient's cells to cure a genetic disease, for example, inserting a working copy of a gene that does not work because of a mutation.

genetic counselor. A professional with a graduate degree in genetic counseling who specializes in genetic disorders and their implications for an individual and his or her family.

geneticist. A scientist who studies genetics or a physician who specializes in the treatment of people with genetic disorders.

heart failure. A medical condition in which the heart cannot pump blood effectively to the body. It can be caused by various diseases.

hemangioma. A benign blood vessel malformation that can occur in various parts of the body.

hematocrit. A measurement of the percentage of red blood cells in the blood.

hemiparesis. Weakness on one side of the body, often caused by a stroke or brain injury.

hemoglobin. The substance in the blood that carries oxygen from the lungs to various parts of the body.

hemoptysis. Coughing up blood.

hemorrhage. Bleeding. The term is usually used to describe excessive bleeding.

hemorrhagic. Caused by or contributing to hemorrhage.

hepatic encephalopathy. A condition caused by advanced liver disease, marked by disturbances of consciousness that may be progressive.

hereditary. Transmitted from one generation to the next through the genes.

HHT Foundation International. See **Cure HHT.**

HHT type 1. HHT caused by mutation in the endoglin (*ENG*) gene.

HHT type 2. HHT caused by mutation in the *ALK1* gene.

high-output heart failure. Heart failure caused by excessive blood flow to the heart, which makes the heart work harder and eventually results in loss of heart function.

hormone. Naturally occurring chemical substance formed by the body and carried to another area where it has a specific effect. Hormones can also be manufactured and administered.

Human Genome Project. A world project designed to locate all the genes of the human body.

human subject. A living person who voluntarily participates in research. The investigator conducting the research collects data about the person through questionnaires, observations of behavior, or interviews or from medical records and/or through experimental medications or procedures.

hypoxemia. A condition in which the amount of oxygen in the blood is reduced.

inflammation. The reaction of living tissue to an injury or infection, characterized by heat, redness, swelling, and pain. HHT research is looking at the role of inflammation as a trigger for AVM growth.

infusion. Slow, continuous introduction of medication through an intravenous drip, e.g., an iron infusion.

interventional radiologist. A doctor specializing in the use of imaging technologies to assist and guide invasive procedures.

intracranial. Located within the brain.

intravenous (IV). Entering the body through a vein.

iron. A metal that is essential for making hemoglobin.

iron deficiency. A condition in which the body does not have enough iron. This can lead to anemia.

iron supplements. Pills or liquid containing iron that can be taken to treat iron deficiency.

juvenile polyposis. A disease marked by multiple polyps in the intestine and increased risk of colon cancer. One of the genes that causes HHT, *SMAD4*, also results in juvenile polyposis.

knock-out mouse. A mouse in which a gene has been inactivated. This type of mouse is used in medical research.

laser photocoagulation. Use of a laser light beam to treat telangiectasias in HHT.

laser therapy. Therapy in which a very intense beam of light is focused on the affected area to treat telangiectasias of the skin, GI tract, and nose.

lesion. An abnormality in an organ of the body. An AVM is a type of lesion.

melena. Black stool resulting from bleeding in the stomach or the duodenum. It may also be caused by oral iron therapy.

migraine. A type of severe headache often preceded by changes in vision (aura). They are more common in patients with HHT who have lung AVMs.

modifier gene. A gene that influences the expression of ("turns on" or "turns off") a different gene.

morbidity. Significant symptoms or complications from a disease or a treatment.

mouse model. See **animal model.**

MRI (magnetic resonance imaging). A scan of the brain (or other organ) that uses magnetic energy to determine the presence of AVMs, aneurysms, stroke, and brain abscess.

mucosa. See **mucous membrane.**

mucous membrane. The membrane that lines body passages and cavities (such as the digestive, respiratory, and genitourinary tracts) that connect directly or indirectly with the outside of the body.

mutation. A change in the genetic code of a gene, which can cause a genetic disorder.

nasal septum. See **septum.**

neurologist. A doctor who specializes in disorders of the nervous system.

neuroradiologist. A radiologist who specializes in the use of radioactive substances (contrast material), x-rays, and scanning devices for the diagnosis and treatment of diseases of the nervous system, including the brain and spinal cord.

neurosurgeon. A surgeon who treats diseases of the brain and nervous system.

nidus. The tangle of blood vessels that forms an AVM.

occlude. To close or block.

occult blood. Blood that is present in the stool but not visible to the eye. Laboratory tests may be used to check for occult blood.

otolaryngologist. See **ENT.**

oxymetazoline. A medication that treats nasal congestion by constricting the blood vessels. It can be used to treat mild nosebleeds.

PAVM (pulmonary arteriovenous malformation). Direct connection between the arteries and veins in the lung.

perforation. A hole, e.g., a perforation of the nasal septum or gut wall.

placebo. A pill or other substance that has no medical effect but may make a person feel better. Placebos are often used in research testing the effectiveness of medications.

pomalidomide. A cancer drug that inhibits blood vessel growth. It is currently being studied to test its use in controlling bleeding in HHT.

portal hypertension. High blood pressure in the portal (liver) vein, which can result from shunting of blood due to liver AVMs.

prophylactic. Preventative; used to prevent a disease or medical problem.

pulmonary. In or having to do with the lungs, e.g., a pulmonary AVM.

pulmonary arterial hypertension. A type of pulmonary hypertension caused by narrowing and stiffening of arteries in the lungs.

pulmonary hypertension. A medical condition in which there is high blood pressure inside the lungs.

radiologist. A doctor who specializes in the use of x-rays or other body imaging techniques.

radiosurgery. See **stereotactic radiation therapy.**

recanalization. The process of blood vessel regrowth and return of blood flow through a previously coiled or plugged AVM.

reperfusion. The process of restoring blood flow to an area where it was blocked or limited.

reticulocyte. A young (newly formed) red blood cell.

sclerotherapy. A treatment for nosebleeds in which an irritating substance is injected directly into blood vessels in the nose, causing scarring that eliminates telangiectasias.

screening. Tests performed to determine the presence of an abnormality or illness before it causes a problem. In HHT, screening is used most often to detect asymptomatic lung and brain AVMs. See also **CAT scan; echo bubble test; MRI.**

septal dermoplasty. A skin graft performed inside the nose to prevent nosebleeds.

septum. The wall of cartilage that divides the nose into two sides.

shunt. The passage of blood directly from an artery to a vein when capillaries are missing.

SMAD4. The gene known to cause HHT and juvenile polyposis.

stereotactic radiation therapy. Therapy in which a metal frame is placed around the skull and a focused x-ray beam is used to try to shrink an AVM of the brain while avoiding injury to the surrounding normal brain.

stroke. A sudden loss of blood supply to the brain, resulting in damage to brain tissue. Stroke symptoms include weakness, numbness, difficulty speaking, and changes in the level of consciousness. Strokes may occur in HHT as a result of a brain AVM bleed or a clot that escapes filtering by the lungs because of a lung AVM. See also **TIA.**

systemic. Affecting the entire body (as opposed to only one area of the body).

telangiectasia. An abnormal connection between small arteries and veins occurring in the gut, mouth, nose (i.e., in the mucosa), or on the skin, where they appear as red or purple spots. It is a small version of an AVM.

TIA (transient ischemic attack). A neurological event with strokelike symptoms that lasts less than 24 hours. See also **stroke.**

tranexamic acid. See **Amicar.**

varices. Enlarged blood vessels in the esophagus that are prone to bleeding, caused by liver failure.

vascular. Referring to or describing blood vessels.

Young's procedure. A surgical procedure that closes the nostrils to treat severe nosebleeds.

Resources

General Information

Organizations

Cure HHT
HHT Foundation International, Inc.
PO Box 329
Monkton, MD 21111 USA
Phone: 410-357-9932
Fax: 410-357-0655
Website: www.curehht.org

NORD
National Organization for Rare Disorders
National Headquarters
55 Kenosia Avenue
Danbury, CT 06810
Phone: 203-744-0100
Fax: 203-798-2291
Website: www.rarediseases.org

E-book

Hereditary Hemorrhagic Telangiectasia: An Overview for Patients and Families, by Scott Olitsky, February 27, 2011. Available in Kindle edition at www.amazon .com. This short e-book summarizes the basics of HHT diagnosis, treatment, and management.

Media Articles

"Against all Odds," by Pam Frampton, *Telegram* (St. John's, NL), May 7, 2016. Available online at http://www.thetelegram.com/Opinion/Columnists/2016 -05-07/article-4521039/Pam-Frampton%3A-Against-all-odds/1.

"Iowa City woman works to raise awareness of rare bleeding disorder," by Alison Gowans, *Cedar Rapids (IA) Gazette*, December 4, 2015. Available online

at http://www.thegazette.com/subject/news/health/iowa-city-woman-works
-to-raise-awareness-of-rare-bleeding-disorder-20151204.

"Mother and infant son fight rare bleeding disorder," by Heather Simonsen,
KSL TV, April 11, 2016. Available online at http://www.ksl.com/?sid
=39286644&nid=148&title=mother-and-infant-son-fight-rare-bleeding
-disorder.

"When a Bloody Nose Is Cause for Concern: Abnormal bleeding may point to
the rare illness HHT." Available online at https://health.clevelandclinic.org
/2015/12/bloody-nose-cause-concern/.

HHT Fact Sheets

The following fact sheets, developed by Cure HHT in collaboration with
experts in medicine, psychology, and genetics, are available to read and
download free at http://curehht.org/resources/hht-brochures/.

Advice for People Newly Diagnosed
   with HHT
Aging Patients with HHT
Coping with HHT: For Teens
Family Ties: Genetic Testing
HHT & Depression

HHT & Stroke
I Have HHT: For Kids
Know the Signs & Symptoms
Living with HHT
My Child Has HHT: Screening Guidelines
My Partner Has HHT

Communicating with Your Doctor

The following fact sheets, developed by Cure HHT in collaboration with
experts in medicine, psychology, and genetics, are available to read and
download free at http://curehht.org/resources/hht-brochures/.
HHT Quick Facts for Health Care Professionals
Talking To Your Physician about HHT

Screening and Treatment: HHT Centers of Excellence

United States

Arkansas

University of Arkansas for Medical Sciences HHT Center
Division of Interventional Radiology
4301 W. Markham Street, #556
Little Rock, AR 72205-7199
Website: http://uamshealth.com/medicalservices/radiology
   /interventionalradiology/hht/
Contact: Paige Womble, RN

Phone: 501-686-6918
Fax: 501-686-8420
Dr. Mollie Meek, Director

California

University of California at Los Angeles HHT Center
UCLA Radiology Consultation Center
100 Medical Plaza, Suite 100
Los Angeles, CA 90095
Website: http://radiology.ucla.edu/hht /
Contact: HHT Center Administrator / Barbara Quinn, Nurse Practitioner
Phone: 310-481-7545
Dr. Justin McWilliams, Codirector
Dr. Gary Duckwiler, Codirector

University of California at San Diego HHT Center
UCSD Medical Center
200 West Arbor Drive, #8756
San Diego, CA 92103
Contact: Julie Fisher, HHT Clinic Coordinator
Phone: 619-543-7965 or 619-543-5670
Dr. Thomas Kinney, Director

University Of California at San Francisco HHT Center
Adult Clinic
185 Berry Street, Suite 180, Lobby 6
San Francisco, CA 94107-0946
Pediatric Clinic
UCSF Ron Conway Family Gateway Medical Building, 5th Floor, Reception
area 5A
UCSF Medical Center at Mission Bay
1825 Fourth Street
San Francisco, CA 94158
Website: https://radiology.ucsf.edu/patient-care/services/specialty-imaging/
Contact: Anjuli Figueira, Patient Care Coordinator
Phone: 415-353-8867
Fax: 415-353-3158
Dr. Miles Conrad, Codirector
Dr. Steven Hetts, Codirector

Colorado

University of Colorado Hospital

12605 E. 16th Avenue
Aurora, CO 80045
Website: https://www.uchealth.org/Pages/OHAM/OrgUnitDetails.aspx
?OrganizationalUnitId=36
Contact: HHT Patient Access Representative
Phone: 720-848-5182
Dr. Brian Graham, Codirector
Dr. Paul Rochon, Codirector

Connecticut

Yale University HHT Center
Department of Diagnostic Radiology
PO Box 208042
789 Howard Avenue, Room CB225
New Haven, CT 06520
Website: http://hht.yale.edu/
Contact: Kate Henderson, MS, CGC
Phone: 203-737-5395
Fax: 203-737-5394
Jeffrey Pollak, MD, Medical Director
Katharine Henderson, MS, CGC, Codirector
Robert I. White Jr., MD, Medical Director Emeritus

Georgia

Augusta University HHT Center
(Formerly Georgia Regents University)
Division of Pulmonary Medicine
1120 15th Street, BBR 5513
Augusta, GA 30912-3135
Website: http://www.augusta.edu/mcg/medicine/pulmonary/pvd/hht/
Contact: Janie Sims, RN
Phone: 706-721-0470
Fax: 706-721-2568
Dr. James Gossage, Director

Illinois

University of Chicago Medicine HHT Center
5841 S. Maryland Avenue, J325
Chicago, IL 60637
Website: http://www.uchospitals.edu/specialties/hht/
Contact: Shannon Love, RN, BSN

Phone: 773-702-4452
Fax: 773-702-3518
Dr. Issam Awad, Director

Maryland

Johns Hopkins HHT Center
Radiology and Radiological Science
Bloomberg 3287
1800 Orleans Street
Baltimore, MD 21287-4010
Website: http://www.hopkinsmedicine.org/interventional-radiology/hht/
Contact: Courtney Myles-Ross
Phone: 410-550-5864
Fax: 410-367-2325
Dr. Christian Merlo, Codirector
Dr. Sally Mitchell, Codirector

Massachusetts

Massachusetts General Hospital (MGH) HHT Center
(Includes affiliations with Massachusetts General Hospital, Massachusetts
General Hospital for Children, and Massachusetts Eye & Ear Infirmary)
Pulmonary Hypertension Clinic
55 Fruit Street, Bulfinch 148
Boston, MA 02114
Website: http://www.massgeneral.org/children/services/treatmentprograms
.aspx?id=1766
Phone: 617-724-3705
Dr. Josanna Rodriguez-Lopez, Codirector
Dr. Ray Liu, Codirector

Minnesota

Mayo Clinic HHT Center
Division of Pulmonary & Critical Care Medicine
200 First Street S.W.
Rochester, MN 55905
Website: http://www.mayoclinic.org/diseases-conditions/hht/hht-care-at
-mayo-clinic/ovc-20170118
Contact: Keri Jacobson, Medical Secretary
Phone: 507-284-2158
Fax: 507-266-4372
Dr. Michael Krowka, Director

Missouri

Washington University HHT Center
660 South Euclid Avenue, #8052
St. Louis, MO 63110-1093
Contact: Dr. Murali Chakinala, Codirector (Adults)
Phone: 877-888-5864 or 314-454-8917
Contact: Dr. Andy White, Codirector (Pediatrics)
Phone: 314-454-2479
Contact: Dr. Jay Piccirillo (ENT)
Phone: 314-362-8641

New York

New York Presbyterian / Columbia University HHT Center
177 Fort Washington Avenue
MBH 4-100
New York, NY 10032
Appointments: 212-326-8874
Dr. Sophie Chheang, Codirector
Dr. David Sperling, Codirector

North Carolina

University of North Carolina at Chapel Hill HHT Center
UNC at Chapel Hill
Department of Hematology
6340 Quadrangle Drive, Suite 50
Chapel Hill, NC 27517
Website: http://www.med.unc.edu/hhtcenter
Contact: Karen Smith, RN
Phone: 919-966-2790
Dr. Raj Kasthuri, Director

Ohio

Cincinnati HHT Center
3333 Burnet Avenue
Cincinnati, OH 44195
Contact: Melissa Morris, Patient Coordinator
Phone: 513-636-2084
Website: https://www.cincinnatichildrens.org/service/h/hereditary
-hemorrhagic-telangiectasia
Dr. Adrienne Hammill, Director
Dr. Manish Patel, Associate Director

Cleveland Clinic HHT Center
9500 Euclid Avenue
Cleveland, OH 44195
Contact: Kasi Timmerman
Phone: 216-445-3636
Fax: 216-636-2054
Dr. Joseph Parambil, Director

Oregon

Oregon Health & Science University HHT Center
OHSU L-605
3181 S.W. Sam Jackson Park Road
Portland, OR 97239
Website: http://www.ohsu.edu/hht/
Contact: Tami Karjalainene
Phone: 503-494-7660 (ext. 1 for HHT Clinic)
Dr. Mark Chesnutt, Director

Pennsylvania

University of Pennsylvania HHT Center
Division of Medical Genetics
3400 Spruce Street, 1115 Penn Tower
Philadelphia, PA 19104-4283
Contact: Meredith Breen
Phone: 215-662-4740
Fax: 215-614-0298
Dr. Reed Pyeritz, Codirector
Dr. Scott Trerotola, Codirector

UPMC and University of Pittsburgh HHT Center
UPMC Presbyterian–Shadyside
200 Lothrop Street
Pittsburgh, PA 15213
Contact: General Call Center (request a referral to the UPMC HHT Center)
Phone: 412-648-6161
Dr. Christopher Faber, Director

Texas

University of Texas–Southwestern HHT Center
University of Texas Southwestern Medical School
5939 Harry Hines Boulevard
Professional Office Building 2, Suite 630

Dallas, TX 75390-9198
Website: http://www.utswmedicine.org/conditionsspecialties/radiology
   /interventional/endovascular-therapy/hht.html
Contact: Vanessa Jimenez
Phone: 214-645-5750
Vicki Diaz, Scheduler
Phone: 214-645-2100
Dr. John Battaile, Director

Utah

University of Utah Medical Center HHT Center
30 North 1900 East
HHT Clinic/1A71
Salt Lake City, UT 84132
Website: http://healthcare.utah.edu/hht/
Contact: HHT Care Coordinator
Phone: 801-581-8188
Fax: 801-581-2414
E-mail: UoUHHT@hsc.utah.edu
Jamie McDonald, MS, CGC, Codirector
Dr. Kevin Whitehead, Codirector

Wisconsin

Froedtert & Medical College of Wisconsin HHT Center
9200 West Wisconsin Avenue
Milwaukee, WI 53226
Website: http://www.froedtert.com/hht
Contact: Jule Meddaugh
Phone: 414-805-3666 or 800-362-8677
Fax: 414-805-3905
Dr. Robert Krippendorf, Director

Canada

Alberta

Edmonton HHT Centre
University of Alberta
3-105C Clinical Sciences Building
Edmonton, AB T6G 2G3
Canada
Phone: 780-492-5879
Fax: 780-492-6739

Dr. Dilini Vethanayagam, Codirector
Dr. Richard Owen, Codirector

Ontario

Toronto HHT Centre
St. Michael's Hospital
30 Bond Street, Room 6049
Toronto, ON M5B 1W8
Canada
Adult HHT & Pulmonary AVM Center
Contact: Rose Pantalone for Dr. Marie Faughnan, Director
Phone: 416-864-6060, ext. 2407
Pediatric HHT Clinic
Director: Dr. Felix Ratjen, Pediatric Respirologist
Hospital for Sick Children
Contact: Susan Carpenter
Phone: 416-813-5837
HHT Genetics Team
The Hospital for Sick Children
Division of Clinical & Metabolic Genetics
555 University Avenue
Toronto, ON M5G1X8
Canada
Website: www.hhttoronto.com
Contact: Ms. Regan Klatt, MS, CGC, Vice-Director
Phone: 416-813-6389
Fax: 416-813-5345
Brain AVM Clinic
University Health Network
Dr. Karel terBrugge, Interventional Neuroradiologist
Phone: 416-603-5266
Brain AVM Study Clinic
Website: http://brainavm.uhnres.utoronto.ca/index.html
Brain AVM Support Group
Website: http://brainavm.uhnres.utoronto.ca/support_group/index.htm

Montreal HHT Centre
CHUM, Hotel Dieu
3840 St-Urbain
Montreal, QC H2W 1T8
Canada
Contact: Anouk Gackowski for Dr. Andreanne Gauthier, Director

Phone: 514-890-8000, ext. 15672
Fax: 514-412-7123
Patient Support Group
Website: http://hhtcanada.com
Isabelle Choquet-Goulet, President

International

There are 22 HHT Centers of Excellence in various countries around the world. A list of these centers can be found on the Cure HHT website at http://curehht.org/resources/hht-treatment-centers/international-2/.

Genetic Counseling

Most HHT Centers of Excellence provide genetic counseling. These are additional resources.

National Society of Genetic Counselors
330 N. Wabash Avenue, Suite 2000
Chicago, IL 60611
Phone: 312-321-6834
Website: www.nsgc.org

American Board of Genetic Counseling
Executive Office
PO Box 14216
Lenexa, KS 66285-4216
Phone: 913-222-8661
Fax: 913-222-8606
Website: www.abgc.net

Genetic Testing Laboratories

Genetic testing must be ordered by a genetic counselor or physician. You can get an order for testing from these labs from your HHT Center of Excellence physician, medical geneticist, genetic counselor, or other physician.

United States

Ambry Genetics
15 Argonaut
Aliso Viejo, CA 92656
Phone: 949-900-5500 or 866-262-7943
Fax: 949-900-5501
E-mail: HHT@ambrygen.com

ARUP Laboratories
500 Chipeta Way
Salt Lake City, UT 84108-1221
Contact: Ms. Jamie McDonald, MS, CGC
Phone: 800-242-2787, ext. 3179
Website: http://www.aruplab.com

Mayo Medical Laboratories
3050 Superior Drive NW
Rochester, MN 55901
Contact: Kate Kotzer, MS, CGC
Phone: 800-533-1710
Website: http://www.mayomedicallaboratories.com

University of Pennsylvania
Genetic Diagnostic Laboratory
Department of Genetics
415 Anatomy-Chemistry Building
3620 Hamilton Walk
Philadelphia, PA 19104-6145
Contact: Jessica Ebrahimzadeh
Phone: 215-573-9161
Fax: 215-573-5940
E-mail: gdllab@mail.med.upenn.edu
Website: http://www.med.upenn.edu/gdl

Canada

Impact Genetics
1100 Bennett Road, Unit 4
Bowmanville, ON L1C 3K5
Canada
Contact: Jeanne McKay
Phone: 877-624-9769
E-mail: info@impactgenetics.com
Website: http://impactgenetics.com

Molecular Genetics Laboratory
The Hospital for Sick Children
555 University Avenue
Roy C. Hill Wing, Room 3-421
Toronto, ON M5G 1X8
Canada

Phone: 416-813-6590
Fax: 416-813-7732
Website: http://www.sickkids.ca/molecular/

International

A list of genetic testing laboratories around the world can be found on the Cure HHT website at http://curehht.org/living-with-hht/genetic-testing/international-genetic-testing-labs/.

Support

HHT Facebook Groups

Cure HHT
Hereditary Hemorrhagic Telangiectasia (HHT) Awareness
HHT Canada THH
HHT in Australia
HHT International
HHT Ireland
HHT—Our Hope Holds the Cure
HHT UK Friends
New Treatments for HHT
Women with HHT

Stroke Support

American Heart Association / American Stroke Association
7272 Greenville Avenue
Dallas, TX 75231
Phone: 800-242-8721
Website: www.strokeassociation.org
Information on stroke causes, recovery, prevention, and support.

Heart and Stroke Association of Canada
Website: www.heartandstroke.ca

National Stroke Association
9707 East Easter Lane, Building B
Englewood, CO 80112
Phone: 800-787-6537
Website: www.stroke.org
Information on all aspects of stroke and recovery, including a list of stroke clubs around the United States.

Pulmonary Hypertension Support

Pulmonary Hypertension Association
801 Roeder Road, Suite 1000
Silver Spring, MD 20910
Phone: 301-565-3004
Website: www.phassociation.org/
Information and support for living with pulmonary hypertension.

Hereditary Hemorrhagic Telangiectasia and PH, pamphlet published by Cure HHT.
Available online at http://curehht.org/wp-content/uploads/2016/02/PH_and
_HHT-PATIENT_Brochure.pdf.

Liver Transplant Support

American Liver Foundation
39 Broadway, Suite 2700
New York, NY 10006
Phone: 212-668-1000
Website: www.liverfoundation.org
Information and a variety of support services and referrals for people who
have liver disease, are anticipating a liver transplant, or are living with a
transplanted liver.

National Institutes of Health
Website: www.niddk.nih.gov/health-information/health-topics/liver-disease
/liver-transplant/Pages/facts.aspx
Provides detailed explanations on liver disease, transplant procedures, and
recovery from transplant surgery.

Heart Failure Support

American Heart Association
7272 Greenville Avenue
Dallas, TX 75231
Phone: 800-242-8721
Website: www.heart.org

Juvenile Polyposis Support

Hereditary Colon Cancer Foundation
1776 Park Avenue, Suite 4-203
Park City, UT 84060
Website: www.HereditaryColonCancerFoundation.org

Support for Family Caregivers

Family Caregiver Alliance
180 Montgomery Street, Suite 1100
San Francisco, CA 94104
Phone: 800-445-8106
Website: www.caregiver.org
Family Caregiving 101
Website: www.familycaregiving101.org

National Alliance for Caregiving
4720 Montgomery Lane, 5th Floor
Bethesda, MD 20814
Website: www.caregiving.org

National Family Caregivers Association
10605 Concord Street, Suite 501
Kensington, MD 20895-2504
Phone: 800-896-3650
Website: www.thefamilycaregiver.org

Rosalynn Carter Institute for Human Development
800 Wheatley Street
Americus, GA 31709
Phone: 229-928-1234
Website: www.rci.gsw.edu
Promotes research, education, training, and advocacy for caregiver issues.

Mental Health Professionals and Family Therapists

American Association of Marriage and Family Therapists
112 South Alfred Street
Alexandria, VA 22314-3061
Phone: 703-838-9808
Provides a therapist-locator service to help with finding a qualified marriage therapist in your local area (www.therapistlocator.net).

American Psychiatric Association
1000 Wilson Boulevard, Suite 1825
Arlington, VA 22209
Phone: 800-357-7924
Website: www.psych.org

National Association of Social Workers
750 First Street NE, Suite 700

Washington, DC 20002
Phone: 202-408-8600
Website: www.socialworkers.org

Disabilty and Insurance Benefits

Centers for Medicare and Medicaid Services (CMS)
US Department of Health and Human Services
Website: www.cms.hhs.gov
Information on Medicare and Medicaid benefits and programs, the Medicaid
waiver, and other programs and services provided by these government health
insurance programs.

Medicare
Phone: 800-633-4227
Website: www.medicare.gov

Social Security Administration
Website: www.ssa.gov
Information on Social Security disability and retirement benefits, the application process, and locating your local Social Security office.

US Department of Veterans Affairs
Federal Benefits for Veterans, Dependants, and Survivors
Website: www.va.gov/

A Shoppers Guide to Long Term Care Insurance, pamphlet published by the
National Association of Insurance Commissioners, 120 W. 12th Street, Suite
100, Kansas City, MO 64105, phone: 816-842-3600. Available online at www
.naic.org.

National Association of Insurance Commissioners
Central Office
1100 Walnut Street, Suite 1500
Kansas City, MO 64106-2197
Phone: 816-842-3600
Website: www.naic.org/documents/members_membershiplist.pdf

Long-Term Care Planning

National Clearinghouse for Long Term Care Information
US Department of Health and Human Services
Website: www.longtermcare.gov

Certified Financial Planner Board of Standards
1425 K Street, NW, Suite 500

Washington, DC 20005
Phone: 800-487-1497
Website: www.cfp.net

This is the board that certifies financial planners. The website provides a locator service for finding a certified financial planner in your local area.

Elder Law Answers
260 West Exchange Street
Suite 004, Box 29
Providence, RI 02903
Phone: 866-267-0947
Website: www.elderlawanswers.com
Information on long-term care, insurance, advance directives; elder care lawyers by location.

Index

Epistaxis Severity Score, 40–41, 134,
145; health problems with, 45; HHT
diagnosis and, 17, 18–19, 20, 21, 22,
23–24, 33, 53, 71, 99–100; juvenile
polyposis and, 72; prevalence, 3, 32;
quality-of-life effects, 138; triggers,
43; work accommodations, 83
nosebleed management, 30, 41–45; by
children, 6, 44–45; how to stop a
nosebleed, 41–42; making a plan
with doctor, 42–43; planning ahead,
43; for social effects, 43–44, 138
nosebleed prevention and treatment,
32, 37–40, 68, 120–21; anti-VEGF
drugs, 135–36; bazedoxifene, 136;
bevacizumab, 37–38, 134, 139;
cauterization, 23, 32, 38, 154, 155;
cold ablation, 38, 154; embolization,
38–39; estriol, 134; estrogen cream,
37; laser therapy, 38, 43, 120, 135;
moisturizers, 37; oxymetazoline,
158; pomalidomide, 139; sclerotherapy, 38, 159; septal dermoplasty, 39,
159; tamoxifen, 136; timolol nose
spray, 140; topical treatments,
134–35, 145; tranexamic acid, 37,
134, 136; Young's procedure, 39,
120, 159
nose telangiectasias, 16, 33, 37–38;
treatments, 38–41, 134–36, 140,
154, 157, 159

Osler, William, 1
Osler-Weber-Rendu syndrome, 2
Our HHT Registry, 142–43
outcomes registry, 6, 142–43
oxygen levels, 18, 20, 22, 33, 81, 155,
157; anemia and, 47, 48, 49; arterial
blood gas test, 153; biliary ischemia
and, 69, 154; hemoglobin and, 47,
156; lung AVMs and, 51, 53, 56, 57,
58, 132; pulmonary hypertension
and, 71
oxygen supplementation, 51, 56
oxymetazoline, 42, 158

parents/parenting, 8, 9, 11, 74, 75, 97,
115; advocating for child with HHT,
111–12; of child with HHT, 108–13;
deciding to become a parent, 105–8;
fostering a positive attitude, 112–13;
guilty feelings, 101; teaching child
about HHT, 110–11. See also family
pazopanib, 140
penicillin, 60
perforation, 46, 158
petroleum jelly, nasal, 37, 134
pilot studies, 133
placebo, 133, 134, 135, 136, 139, 144,
146, 158
pomalidomide, 46, 139–40, 158
portal hypertension, 68–69, 158
positive attitude, 79, 80, 87–89, 90,
102, 108, 112–13
pregnancy: IVF and, 106–7; lung AVMs
in, 51; nosebleeds in, 7; prenatal
genetic testing, 29, 106–8; termination of, 107
preimplantation genetic diagnosis
(PGD), 107, 108
priority setting, 81, 112
pulmonary angiography, 57
pulmonary arterial hypertension
(PAH), 70–71, 158
pulmonary AVMs (PAVMs). See lung
AVMs
pulmonary hypertension (PH), 10, 68,
70–72, 74, 81, 158, 173; screening,
71–72, 155; treatment, 72
Pulmonary Hypertension Association,
74, 173
pulse oximetry, 53, 55, 58

quality of life, 10, 49, 79, 80, 115, 127,
138–39; Avastin and, 135, 139;
timolol and, 140

race/ethnicity, 3
radiosurgery, 65, 158
randomized controlled trials (RCTs),
133, 134, 135, 136, 139, 144